Natural Treatments
for Tics & Tourette's

Natural Treatments for Tics & Tourette's

A PATIENT AND FAMILY GUIDE

Sheila J. Rogers

North Atlantic Books
Berkeley, California

ASSOCIATION FOR COMPREHENSIVE NEUROTHERAPY
Broken Arrow, Oklahoma
WWW.TicsAndTourettes.com

Published by the Association for Comprehensive NeuroTherapy
P.O. Box 210848
Royal Palm Beach, FL 33421-0848
and
North Atlantic Books
P.O. Box 12327
Berkeley, California 94712

Cover design by Claudia Smelser
Book layout by Sandy Glassman
Printed in the United States of America

Disclaimer: The material in this book is for educational purposes only and is not intended as specific treatment recommendations for individuals or as medical advice. The suggestions in this book are not intended as a substitute for consulting with a physician. No product, practice, or practitioner mentioned in this book is being endorsed. The purpose of this book is not to advise whether a particular therapy should be used. Neither the editor, authors of articles, the Association for Comprehensive NeuroTherapy and its board members, *Latitudes* and its professional advisory board, publisher, distributors, nor any related party make any claims regarding the effects of the therapies and approaches discussed; they cannot accept legal responsibility for any approach or treatment undertaken. Please consult a qualified health care practitioner for appropriate treatment.

Natural Treatments for Tics & Tourette's is sponsored by the Society for the Study of Native Arts and Sciences, a nonprofit educational corporation whose goals are to develop an educational and cross-cultural perspective linking various scientific, social, and artistic fields; to nurture a holistic view of arts, sciences, humanities, and healing; and to publish and distribute literature on the relationship of mind, body, and nature.

North Atlantic Books' publications are available through most bookstores. For further information, visit our website at www.northatlanticbooks.com or call 800-733-3000.

Library of Congress Cataloging-in-Publication Data

Rogers, Sheila J. 1948–
   Natural treatments for tics and tourette's : a patient and family guide /
Sheila J. Rogers.
      p. cm.
   Includes bibliographical references.
   ISBN 978-1-55643-747-2
   1. Tourette syndrome. 2. Tourette syndrome—Alternative treatment.
3. Tic disorders. 4. Tic disorders—Alternative treatment. I. Title.
   RC375.R638 2008
   616.8'3—dc22
                                                2008025395

   5 6 7 8 9 10 SHERIDAN 17 16 15 14

Dedicated to Ginger and Griffin Wakem

Contents

Acknowledgments

I GREATLY APPRECIATE THE CONTRIBUTIONS to this book made by professional experts, patients, and family members throughout the global community. Each demonstrated resolve and foresight in investigating new methods of healing for tic disorders. They have shared their findings in the hope of helping others.

The efforts of the advisory board of our organization's publication, *Latitudes,* provided the foundation for *Tics and Tourette's*: John Boyles, MD; Leon Chaitow, ND, DO; Abram Hoffer, MD, PhD; Helen Irlen, MA; Melvin Kaplan, OD; Ricki Linksman, MS; Siegfried Othmer, PhD; Jon Pangborn, PhD; William Philpott, MD; William Rea, MD; Judyth Reichenberg, ND; Bernard Rimland, PhD; Joseph T. Rogers, DO; Sherry Rogers, MD; W. A. Shrader, MD; Dana Ullman, MPH; John E. Upledger, DO; William Walsh, PhD; Mark E. Young, PhD; and Marshall Zaslove, MD. I offer special thanks to board member Albert F. Robbins, DO, who has been my mentor in exploring the benefits of environmental medicine.

Thanks to all who offered their skills in bringing this book to print: Jonathan Kruger, Ed Lee of LeePR, Valerie Tarrant, Sue DeCosmo, Douglas Kruger, Andy Gabor, Ginger Wakem, Steven E. Polyanchek, Annie Lee Leveritt, Herman Fernau, Jean English, Sharan Shively, Alan Yurko, Rick Ma, Larry Teich, Dawn Hess, Chris Phelps-Thiry, Ray Karlin, Kristen Thomas, Cheri Marshall, Bill Phipps, Arthur Stein, and Angela McKenzie. John Steigerwald of Larchmont, New York, has repeatedly raised much-needed funds for ACN through Ironman USA competitions and the Janus Charity Challenge; this book would not have been possible without his dedicated efforts. Sandy Glassman humored me through countless challenges and donated her time to complete the book's layout. And thank you to our manuscript editor, Kimberly L. Hines, who, with a deft hand, brought clarity and freshness to this book.

The ongoing influence of my remarkable parents, Joseph and Sheila Rogers, has helped shape this text. I have also enjoyed the support and counsel of my sister, Lisa, and brothers, Jody and Felix. Lastly, special thanks to my wonderful adult children, Chris, Mona, and Rose. Their volunteer efforts have been invaluable: Chris developed and maintains our organization's website (*www.Latitudes.org*), Mona is our education specialist, and Rose provides advice on graphic arts and environmental issues. Beyond these contributions, their constant support of my driving passion to find safe, natural ways to treat tics and Tourette syndrome, often at the expense of family time and resources, means more to me than they realize.

Introduction

MOST OF US KNOW SOMEONE WITH A CHRONIC muscle tic or twitch that seems a nuisance, but nothing more. On the other hand, some people's tics are so devastatingly serious that daily life is almost unbearable. Regardless of the severity of the tic disorder that concerns you, this book will be helpful and enlightening.

In conventional medicine, mild cases of tics are usually not treated because recommended medications can cause side effects more troublesome than the symptoms themselves. Patients are usually told to simply go home and see whether symptoms improve. When the tics are long-term and include both movement and vocalizations (involuntary noises or words), physicians are likely to diagnose the condition as Tourette syndrome.

Families are often told that Tourette syndrome or other serious tic disorders are genetic and that the use of strong drugs and the reduction of stress are the only helpful approaches. However, many people refuse the medications, or they discontinue them out of dissatisfaction. To date, doctors have had few alternatives to share with patients.

A change for the better!

We invite you to join us as we explore exciting new options for treating tics. The path has already been cleared by determined patients and families and by cutting-edge doctors who were bold enough to break convention and seek better answers. These findings have been compiled for the first time in this text. You will read of successful outcomes from families such as those described next who dealt with symptoms that ranged from mild to severe. Each brought its own form of suffering.

From a woman who struggled with tics throughout her life:
As the years went on, it became increasingly difficult to live with my tic disorder. It was especially embarrassing to have dinner at a restaurant. Just

getting the spoon to my mouth was a horrendous chore.—*A letter to ACN, Chapter 6*

From a father with Tourette syndrome:
I was heartbroken when my six-year-old daughter, Maria, showed signs of the disorder. She then began having more frequent facial tics and also made little noises. I knew too well the challenges that could lie ahead for her. —*"Maria," Chapter 2*

From a mother who battled to help her son:
Aaron started manifesting major tics—such as banging his chin and a whiplash motion of his head and neck, along with many loud vocal tics. Obsessive and compulsive symptoms were also intense.—*"Aaron," Chapter 2*

Medicine operates from a strong paradigm, or framework. The expectation is that observations, findings, and advances will come from its ranks, but occasionally important information is discovered, synthesized, and disseminated by persons outside the formal medical research structure. Such is the case for Ginger Wakem and Marshall Mandell, MD, about whom you will soon read and many others who followed their lead.

Congratulations to you for seeking new avenues in healing. Congratulations also to the children and resolute families described in this book who brought tics and related disorders under control without the use of drugs.

New treatment options

Fortunately, new information takes the treatment of tics to a new level. A growing understanding is emerging of how lifestyle, diet, and the environment, as well as alterations in immune system function can affect symptoms. The research community has shown little interest in nondrug treatments, and for this reason, related studies are often unavailable. Yet, clinicians and patients are now reporting successful interventions for tics without the use of standard medications. This book shares this comprehensive information with the public. You will learn how medical experts and families pursued their own investigations that resulted in these discoveries. Here you will be given the tools you need to begin your own search for help.

How our movement started

This book has its roots in an effort that began in 1986, when a bright and resourceful parent, Ginger Wakem, began an informal network to share information from physicians and patients on nonconventional therapies for tics. Ginger's inspiration for this effort was personal. She had helped her son, Griffin, conquer severe Tourette syndrome without the use of drugs, after regular medications had failed. (See page 36 for the Wakem story.) Ginger assumed physicians who used traditional therapies would be fascinated to learn about her son's dramatic recovery and similar reports from others who used dietary changes, nutritional supplements, and a specialized allergy treatment plan. Instead, she met strong resistance; specialists either ignored her or insisted she was wrong.

The start of *Latitudes* and ACN

At Ginger's request, I stepped in to try to help. I soon found myself in the role of investigative reporter, questioning and documenting the new insights and discoveries in this area. In 1993, I built on Ginger's efforts and launched *Latitudes*, a health publication featuring more than twenty nationally known consultants in the fields of integrative and alternative medicine and later founded an organization built on the same premise. We started by networking with leaders in the field and began aggressively collecting recommendations and case reports related to new ideas for treating tic disorders and

> At Ginger's request, I stepped in to try to help. I soon found myself in the role of investigative reporter, questioning and documenting new insights and discoveries in this area.

Tourette's. This information is now published in *Latitudes Online*, a magazine that continues to be the leading source for up-to-date information on treating tics and accompanying disorders without standard drugs. For more information about this publication, please see page 274.

It soon became a top priority to share these finding with others. From this movement grew the Association for Comprehensive NeuroTherapy (ACN), which was registered as a nonprofit organization in 1996. The name of our group was chosen to reflect the philosophy that therapies for neurologic conditions, or brain disorders, must often be comprehensive to achieve best results; a multidisciplinary approach is often required for true healing to take place.

Groundbreaking survey results

The ACN has been in the forefront of exploring reports about factors that cause tics to increase and alternative approaches that may be used to reduce them.

In Chapter 4, the groundbreaking results of our new ACN Tic Triggers survey are announced. Survey results present the elements that most likely trigger tics, all based on our readers' experience. The survey focused on potential aggravating factors, many of which are as yet unrecognized in the standard literature. Completed by more than 1,790 patients and caregivers, the results provide valuable insight that can help explain what may be aggravating the tics or twitches affecting you or a loved one.

Results of a separate ACN-sponsored survey were recently published in a research journal: "Nutritional Supplements and Complementary/Alternative Medicine in Tourette Syndrome" (*Journal of Child Adolescent Psychopharmacology*; 2004;14:582–89). Results of this survey reinforce the fact that large numbers of people are turning to treatments for tics that do not require drugs, often with good results.

Open-minded collaboration

The information in this book is the culmination of our interaction with talented and dedicated physicians, researchers, holistic practitioners, psychologists, educators, patients, and families. We do not have answers for every person with a tic disorder or an accompanying condition, yet remarkable progress has been made in defining new ways to approach prevention and treatment. More research is needed; however, regardless of the lack of current research, all signs point to even greater progress in the future. Certainly, we are learning more each day.

In an effort to coordinate conventional medical treatments and complementary or alternative approaches, Gerald Erenberg, MD, has offered to serve as liaison between the national Tourette Syndrome Association (TSA)—the lead organization on conventional treatment for Tourette's—and ACN. Dr. Erenberg was chairman of TSA's medical advisory board for many years.

It is now clear that, in many cases, tic conditions can be treated naturally, without the concern for side effects associated with traditional medications.

I invite you to join this important movement by sharing your expertise and experiences with us, particularly your findings after reading this book and trying these ideas. The Association for Comprehensive NeuroTherapy welcomes your input through our website, e-mail, or standard mail. Together we can find the answers needed to overcome the challenges of tic disorders.

Sheila J. Rogers, MS, Director
Association for Comprehensive NeuroTherapy (ACN)
Editor, *Latitudes Online; www.Latitudes.org*
Broken Arrow, Oklahoma

✦

How to Use This Book

Tics and Tourette's contains reports of success in using natural treatments, medical references, and additional resources. Topics include diet and nutritional therapy, allergy and environmental medicine, stress reduction, behavioral and cognitive approaches, homeopathy, biofeedback, immune therapies, osteopathic manipulative treatment and craniosacral therapy, and acupuncture, as well as the use of diagnostic laboratory studies. Techniques that can benefit both mild and serious tic disorders, including Tourette syndrome, are discussed. Most of the approaches can be used along with conventional medication.

You will read the accounts of eleven families who share how they were able to help a member control tics without the use of drugs, and letters from more than 30 others. Each of these examples represents similar successes being experienced by people around the world.

Helping you get the most benefit

In this book, you will encounter a great deal of new information—too much for most people to remember without taking notes. It's a good idea to keep a pen handy in order to jot down your thoughts on the "Notes" sections placed throughout the book.

Most chapters end with a "Take Away Tips" section that highlights some of the key points in the chapter to help you stay focused when implementing interventions. Handy checklists and action plans are also included.

The meaning of "natural" and "alternative"

It is easiest to understand the use of the term *natural* in the book's title by clarifying what it does *not* mean. We use this term to discuss treatments that do not involve the conventional medications typically used to treat tics. Natural treatments have a common function in assisting the body in the healing process. This function contrasts with drug therapies that are used to suppress symptoms.

The terms *alternative, integrative,* and *complementary* are used interchangeably in the text when discussing therapies, because their meanings often overlap or change with time.

Understanding the tic spectrum

Tic disorders range from symptoms that include occasional mild twitching or verbal murmurings to severe and life-altering muscular jerks or vocal outbursts. Please see page 4 for categories of tics, including Tourette syndrome. While it is understandable to want to assign a diagnostic label to the tic symptoms listed on the categories page, it is not always useful from a treatment standpoint. In fact, the Tourette Syndrome Association suggests that the distinction between the different categories "may be no more than semantic."

With this understanding, rather than focusing on which category a particular case of tics falls into, you may find it more beneficial to concentrate on trying to discover what is causing the symptoms to occur and how the problem can be corrected.

As you read this book, bear in mind that you will need to use common sense when considering the options discussed, taking the nature and severity of your situation into account.

When a tic is not a tic

Some tics do not fall into the categories described on page 4. Involuntary muscular movement can be symptomatic of a number of other medical conditions. These include: Huntington's disease, Sydenham's chorea, tremors, tardive dyskinesia, cerebral palsy, Lesch-Nyhan syndrome, restless leg syndrome, dystonias, Wilson's disease, Rett syndrome, Lyme disease, postviral encephalitis, hemiballismus, ataxias, spasmodic torticollis, benign muscle fibrillation, motor neuron diseases, neuroacanthocytosis, endocrine disorders, seizures, thyroid disease, tumors, kidney failure, multiple sclerosis, Parkinson's disease, reactions to medications, and other disorders.

Consultation with a neurologist or other qualified physician is recommended for a definitive diagnosis of muscle tics. The Association for Comprehensive NeuroTherapy's efforts related to tics focus on the disorders listed on page 4.

Practitioner contact information

Contact information for many of the experts included in this text is included in the Appendix. See also Chapter 22 on finding practitioners.

Technical level and repetition

A few chapters written by experts are quite technical, and you will see a note on the opening chapter page to alert you to this shift. Inclusion of this important text provides a scientific basis for many of the practical applications presented. You may wish to share these sections with your physician.

Some themes are repeated across chapters, particularly the role of diet, nutritional supplements, allergy, and environmental medicine. This repetition is purposeful. These are the most commonly reported approaches that patients, families, and physicians have found helpful in treating tics without conventional drugs, and they warrant the most attention. Additional alternative and integrative therapies are also reviewed, with objective reports on their current status in treating tic conditions, to the best of our knowledge. The theme of becoming one's own advocate is also emphasized.

Types of medical reporting presented

There are three levels of medical evidence, and we provide you with relevant information from each of these levels.

The first and highest level or "gold standard" of scientific evidence occurs with a randomized, double-blind, placebo-controlled study. This means that the treatment is assigned in a random manner, that the treatment groups are similar, and that neither the patient nor the doctor (or researcher) knows whether a participant is receiving the active treatment or a placebo. A placebo is similar in appearance to the treatment but is designed to have no effect. Then, results are compared.

The second level of evidence occurs when the research methods include participants who were not selected in a randomized manner or when the study itself is a scientific analysis of outcomes of prospective (looking ahead) or retrospective (looking back) research. An example of a second level of evidence is an epidemiologic survey to determine characteristics, such as the effect of a treatment, within a certain population. This level also includes information received through professional or patient/family checklists and surveys.

The third level represents expert opinion and consensus statements. It may also involve studies of scientific rigor which are conducted on small numbers of participants (pilot studies). It may include case reports, or what is called *anecdotal evidence*. In these instances, a professional or patient/family member describes his or her experience. This is the least objective in the categories of evidence.

In this book, we offer the best available research information. In each instance, we try to find evidence of the highest scientific rank. We also share new survey results from ACN and other sources, provide authoritative recommendations, and give you anecdotal or case report evidence, as appropriate. Most of medicine is based on expert opinion and best practices standards. Evidence-based medicine is a goal that is infrequently achieved.

Common abbreviations and conditions

ACN: The Association for Comprehensive NeuroTherapy, located in Royal Palm Beach, Florida, is the nonprofit organization responsible for the development of this book. The ACN collects and shares information on nondrug treatments for autism, tics and Tourette syndrome, obsessive-compulsive disorder, attention deficit disorder/hyperactivity, depression, anxiety, and learning problems. ACN publishes the subscription magazine *Latitudes Online,* a free e-newsletter *(ACN Today)*, and the blog *"Better Brains, Naturally."* Please see page 274 for more information.

ADHD (and **ADD**): Attention deficit hyperactivity disorder. Three aspects of attention deficit disorder have been identified: (1) inattentive; (2) hyperactive; and (3) impulsive. An individual may have one or more of these aspects. When a person is primarily inattentive, he or she is often said to simply have ADD.

OCD: Obsessive-compulsive disorder. Obsessions are intrusive thoughts, impulses, or images that repeatedly occur. Although the individual realizes that these thoughts may be illogical, he or she feels unable to control them. Compulsions are the acts a person performs in an attempt to deal with obsessions. For example, one might need his window blinds to be "just so" before he can go to sleep and, therefore, spends hours adjusting them, although he is exhausted. We all deal with these issues to some degree; we may check the stove a couple of times before leaving home just to be sure it is turned off. It is when the thoughts or acts become excessive and troublesome that a clinician may diagnose the condition as OCD. The symptoms can be so severe that they are traumatic and disabling.

TS or Tourette's: Tourette syndrome. See page 4 and Chapter 1 for an overview of this condition.

PANDAS: Pediatric autoimmune neuropsychiatric disorders associated with streptococcal infection. See pages 13–15 and Chapter 15.

References and resources

Please refer to the Appendix for lists of related organizations and agencies, scientific references, and recommended reading.

SECTION ONE

Addressing the Causes and Current Treatment of Tics

CHAPTER

1

An Overview of Tic Disorders

IF YOU ARE CONCERNED ABOUT TICS in yourself or someone you care about, you are in good company. The incidence of tics has skyrocketed alarmingly over the last few decades, particularly in Western countries.

An article in *Current Opinion in Neurology* (2003) described the tic disorder known as Tourette syndrome (TS), once considered rare and unusual, as "common." Temporary or transient tics in childhood were termed "very common." This troubling increased incidence mirrors recent increases in such conditions as autism, attention deficit disorder, hyperactivity, depression and bipolar disorder, obsessive-compulsive disorder, and schizophrenia.

A study in 2001 of schoolchildren in and around Rochester, New York, revealed that nearly 20% of students in elementary through high school had some level of tics. The rate among students in special education classes was 27%. A second study found mild to severe tics in 24% of a student population in Washington, DC. In the United Kingdom, results of a 1997 study showed that 65% of students with serious emotional or behavioral difficulties requiring residential placement had tics, and most of those with tics met the criteria for TS.

Although estimates vary, it seems illogical and irresponsible to simply accept these

Categories of Tics

Transient tic disorders: These usually begin between ages five and ten years and are estimated to affect up to 18% of children in the United States. Facial tics and eye blinking are common; the disorder can also include mild sounds or humming. Occasionally tics are unusual in nature. The tics tend to change over time, with one type of tic being replaced by another. Tic episodes usually last a few weeks or months and are most noticeable during times of stress, excitement, or fatigue. Episodes can recur over a period of several years.

Chronic tic disorders: These tics occur over many years and are relatively unchanging—such as an eye twitch that continues unchanged for years.

Chronic multiple tics: This category is difficult to distinguish from transient and chronic tics. The impression is that of having several chronic tics at once.

Tourette syndrome: This category can be the most debilitating of all tic disorders. It is described as having the following characteristics in the *Diagnostic and Statistical Manual of Mental Disorders IV:*

- Both multiple motor and one or more vocal tics have been present at some time during the illness, although not necessarily concurrently;
- The tics occur many times a day (usually in bouts) nearly every day or intermittently throughout a period of more than one year. During this time, there is never a tic-free period of more than three consecutive months;
- The disturbance causes marked distress or significant impairment in social, occupational, or other important areas of functioning;
- The onset occurs before 18 years; and
- The disturbance is not due to the direct physiological effects of a substance (eg, stimulants) or a general medical condition (eg, Huntington's disease or post viral encephalitis).

"The difference between Tourette syndrome and other tic syndromes may be no more than semantic, especially since recent genetic evidence links Tourette syndrome with multiple and transient tics of childhood and can only be defined in retrospect."

Adapted from *A Physician's Guide to the Diagnosis of Tourette Syndrome;* Tourette Syndrome Association

See also pediatric autoimmune neuropsychiatric disorder associated with group A streptococcal infections (PANDAS), pages 13–15.

growing numbers without investigating causes for these increases. Strangely, the medical community and public have not expressed major concern over this situation, and research has not focused on why such an increase in tics is being seen.

Movements and vocalizations

Patterns and types of tics vary greatly among those dealing with these disorders. The categories of tics listed on the opposite page give an overview of the diagnoses physicians use to categorize patients with tics. Fortunately, most tic symptoms are mild.

Some tic movements, such as sniffing, shoulder shrugs, and neck jerks, are termed *simple* and only involve one muscle group. *Complex* tics, on the other hand, involve movements that use multiple muscle groups with coordinated movement. Examples of complex tics are twirling or jumping while walking, and imitating someone's actions. Tics can occur from head to foot. They can be as mild as an occasional eye blink or severe enough to affect large muscles and knock someone from a chair.

Tics can occur from head to foot. They can be as mild as an occasional eye blink or severe enough to affect large muscles and knock someone from a chair.

A simple motor, or movement tic can be severe in its expression; simple does not imply that the tic has less impact on an individual than a complex tic. Tics can also involve touching others or distressing self-injurious behaviors, such as slapping oneself, playing with sharp objects, or touching hot items. Vocal tics may be barely noticeable: a light cough or hum—yet some are disruptive and embarrassing: a loud shout, yelp, squeal, bark, repeating phrases just heard, or swearing (coprolalia). People often feel a sensory urge to tic that has been described by some as similar to the need to scratch an itch. After ticcing there is a sensation of released tension. The ability to recognize a sensory urge to tic increases with age; children younger than ten years are much less aware of that urge.

A large percentage of people report being able to withhold, or postpone tics for short periods, but the tics are usually "released" later. The ability to sense, or experience an urge to tic allows for this adjustment. Many people with tics become experts at disguising associated movements so they appear natural. For example, a person might appear to brush hair out of the face to make a neck jerk seem intentional. Considerable energy and attention are needed to withhold or disguise tics. Doing so can increase stress and result in physical and emotional fatigue. When children withhold tics during school, they may end up releasing them in an explosive and emotionally stressful manner at home.

Preschool children can have tics, as can elderly individuals. Childhood tics often decrease after adolescence or early adulthood.

Coexisting conditions

In the United States, approximately half of children with TS also have attention deficit disorder with hyperactivity (ADHD). Researchers also estimate that more than half of those with TS have learning problems and/or obsessive-compulsive disorder. Anxiety and panic attacks, separation anxiety, and depression are also common. Behavioral difficulties and mood swings are frequently reported, adding to the difficulty of targeting treatment. Trichotillomania (involuntary hair-pulling) occurs at higher than average rates among those with TS. Sleep problems, bedwetting, and numerous other complaints are also frequently reported. Research suggests that patients with TS have a nearly fourfold increased occurrence of migraine headache compared with the general population.

Dealing with these coexisting conditions can be as difficult for the patient and family as the tics themselves, if not more so. See pages 52–53 for a discussion on the implications of coexisting conditions.

Current thought on tic symptoms

The treatment of tics has undergone dramatic change during the last century. Initially, psychologic dysfunction was thought to be the cause of tic disorders; and, therefore, the therapeutic focus was on counseling and psychotherapy, with disappointing results. Then, in the 1960s, scientists found a medical, or biological basis, for the condition, and clinicians began to prescribe medications to treat the brain and nervous system. This was a major breakthrough and resulted in improved tic control, yet it came with a caveat that remains true today. These medications are strong, often untested in children and may have serious side effects. Therefore, the severity of symptoms and the extent to which they affect quality of life determines whether drugs are advised.

No medical test exists to differentiate most tic conditions, nor can any laboratory work indicate the presence of a tic disorder or TS. At present, scientists theorize that an abnormal metabolism of the neurotransmitter dopamine is one cause. A neurotransmitter is a chemical that transmits or carries a signal from one nerve cell to another. Chemicals are released by one neuron and cross a synapse, or space, before being accepted by the next neuron. This is how nerve impulses "communicate." It is theorized that a problem with the receiving neuron results in excess dopamine in the synapse.

Other neurotransmitters, including serotonin, are also thought to be involved. Primarily, researchers blame genetic makeup for the brain transmitter abnormalities seen with tics. Interestingly, approximately four times as many males have TS as do females, although estimates of this ratio vary.

Although a strong genetic component is probable, finding a single gene responsible for tic disorders does not seem likely despite significant efforts to date. Valuable work by genetics researcher, David E. Comings, MD, author of *Search for the Tourette Syndrome and Human Behavior Genes* (1996), has led to a greater understanding of the interaction of tic disorders with other psychologic or neuropsychiatric conditions.

> Valuable work by genetics researcher, David E. Comings, MD, author of *Search for the Tourette Syndrome and Human Behavior Genes* (1996), has led to a greater understanding of the interaction of tic disorders with other psychologic or neurologic conditions.

Neuroimaging studies—brain mappings—of a population of patients with TS suggest abnormalities in the composition of the basal ganglia and frontal lobe white matter in the brain. The basal ganglia helps prioritize information coming to the brain and is associated with large and small motor movements. When the information being received is not filtered properly as a result of dopamine dysfunction, a range of neuropsychiatric symptoms can result. Research suggests that other areas of the brain may also play a significant role. A dysfunction of the hypothalamus with accompanying dysregulation of heat control in the body has been linked to TS.

The environment's role

Environmental factors are known to be involved in the development of tic symptoms. For example, two identical twins could have the same genetic predisposition for tics, but it is their lifestyles, or experiences that determine how the genes for each twin are expressed.

Thomas M. Hyde, MD, and colleagues completed compelling research on identical twins with at least one of each twin set having TS. They found that genetics alone did not account for the development of or the level of severity of TS. Dr. Hyde suggests that there is an interaction between environmental insults to the central nervous system and the genetic component of TS: "TS is a unique example of a medical condition in which genetic and environmental factors influence cerebral development and function to produce a complex neuropsychiatric disorder."

Research to determine these environmental factors is lacking. Since its founding, ACN has vigorously emphasized the necessity of identifying environmental situations that can influence the development and expression of tics. This book is the first publication to share detailed information on numerous environmental factors that can trigger tics, and guidance is provided on how to address these issues. Far more work is needed to further identify the role of the environment in tic disorders, from conception through daily life.

> Since its founding, ACN has vigorously emphasized the necessity of identifying environmental situations that can influence the development and expression of tics.

Stimulant medications

Researcher G. S. Golden, MD, made the case in 1988 that stimulant drugs such as methylphenidate (Ritalin) can increase the severity of tics in patients with TS and that they may occasionally precipitate or initiate TS in patients who previously did not show symptoms of this disorder. He called for physicians to use a conservative approach in treating children with attention deficit disorders with stimulant medication and recommended that behavior management, environmental manipulation, and reducing stress be tried before considering such medication.

It has been 17 years since Dr. Golden's cautions, and the controversy over the role of stimulants in tic disorders continues. Most researchers agree that stimulant medications can initiate or aggravate tics in some people. In fact, the Tourette Syndrome Association (see page 4) specifies that a diagnosis of Tourette syndrome should ensure that symptoms are "not due to the direct physiological effects of a substance (eg, stimulants)." Other researchers consider the stimulant-tic disorder connection to be an uncommon occurrence.

Side Effects of Standard Medications

Some potential adverse effects of a few drugs that are prescribed for tic disorders when symptoms warrant their use are listed below. The descriptions are greatly abbreviated. This information should not be used for decision-making. A quick review will highlight the urgency of finding better treatments for tics.

ORAP

Pimozide (Orap) is an antipsychotic drug.

- Can impair mental and physical abilities;
- Dry mouth, constipation, drowsiness, sedation, impaired muscle movement, restlessness, agitation, adverse behavior, headache;
- May lower the convulsive threshold for seizures;
- Numerous drug interactions; may cause tumors;
- Parkinson-like symptoms, mild to moderately severe, usually reversible;
- Tardive dyskinesia: potentially irreversible, involuntary movements;
- Changes in electrocardiogram;
- Neuroleptic malignant syndrome: a potentially fatal symptom complex;
- Hyperpyrexia (high body temperature) has been reported with antipsychotic drugs;
- Sudden unexpected deaths have occurred.

HALDOL

Haloperidol (Haldol) is an antipsychotic drug.

- Bronchopneumonia: sometimes fatal;
- Rapid mood swing to depression may occur in those with bipolar condition;
- Difficulty in speaking or swallowing; inability to move eyes;
- Loss of balance control; muscle spasms;
- Restlessness, agitation, anxiety;
- Weight gain or loss;
- May cause tardive dyskinesia and neuroleptic malignant syndrome, as with Orap;
- May lower threshold for seizures;
- Negative cardiovascular effects and impaired liver function; increased body temperature.

CATAPRES

Clonidine hydrochloride (Catapres) helps control high blood pressure.

- Sudden cessation of clonidine treatment may cause nervousness, agitation, headache, and tremor;
- This drug should be used during pregnancy and when nursing only if clearly needed;
- Most adverse effects are mild and may diminish with therapy. The most frequent are: dry mouth, drowsiness, dizziness, constipation and sedation;
- The frequency of central nervous system depression may be higher in children than adults.

TENEX

Guanfacine hydrochloride (Tenex) helps control high blood pressure.

- Drowsiness, especially when first taking it;
- Constipation;
- Dizziness;
- Dry mouth;
- Fatigue, sleepiness;
- Headache;
- Impotence;
- Weakness;
- May feel intoxicated after only a small amount of alcohol;
- Mania and aggression (in patients with attention deficit hyperactivity disorder).

NOTE: These and most other drugs prescribed for tics are not well-tested for children under age 12 years, yet they are often prescribed for this group.

(Source: adapted from *Physician's Desk Reference*/package inserts.)

Recent studies have suggested that the use of stimulants in children in whom a diagnosis of ADHD plus Tourette's has been established will not increase the existing tic symptoms in most patients. A published study concludes that stimulants will not increase the initial risk of developing tics. However, these reports are contrary to popular thought and many clinical observations. Additional research is needed to clarify the issue.

Standard efforts to reduce tics

When the tic disorder is mild and does not significantly interfere with daily life, medication is usually not recommended because of the potential for negative side effects. Some commonly used drugs are neuroleptic agents, such as risperidone (Risperdal), olanzapine (Zyprexa), pimozide (Orap), haloperidol (Haldol), and fluphenazine (Prolixin). Researchers initially developed neuroleptics, or tranquilizers, for treating patients with psychosis; these medications have been "borrowed" for tic therapy.

Another class of drugs used in patients with tic disorders are alpha blockers, such as clonidine hydrochloride (Catapres) and guanfacine (Tenex); they are typically used to treat high blood pressure. Clonazepam (Klonopin), sometimes prescribed for tics, is also used as an anticonvulsant and for reducing anxiety. Baclofen, a muscle relaxant and an antispastic agent used for multiple sclerosis, is being explored for treating patients with TS.

For the benefit of those who are not familiar with the potential side effects of these types of drugs, a summary of some is included on page 9. Information on these and other medications is often available online through the drug manufacturer, the website *www. Drugs.com*, or through consultation with your pharmacist.

Research on Botox, nicotine, and behavioral therapies

In recent years, the practice of injecting botulinum toxin, commonly referred to as Botox, into troublesome tic areas to "freeze" the muscle response has been used. Use of Botox is growing as a new option for tic control, though research results are mixed.

Researchers have also investigated the use of nicotine patches and the antihypertensive drug, mecamylamine (Inversine), which blocks nicotine receptors in the brain. Results suggest that these approaches may help reduce the amount of tic medication needed, particularly haloperidol (Haldol). However, these medications did not appear to be useful when used alone, and side effects were problematic for some who tried the nicotine-related interventions. Archie A. Silver, MD, a lead investigator for this subject, has indicated that nicotine therapy may be useful on an as-needed basis, but long term use is not recommended.

Behavioral therapies for tic disorders have been studied with limited yet promising results. This approach is not often recommended by physicians, and appropriately trained behavior therapists can be difficult to locate. Please see Chapter 20 for more on behavioral therapies.

Cannabis (marijuana) therapy

It has long been reported that marijuana has properties that can help reduce tic symptoms. Legal and political issues have delayed research into this subject. In 2003, a few small studies were conducted on the use of Delta9-tetrahydrocannabinol (THC), the most active ingredient in cannabis, for TS. The product, Marinol, pure synthetic THC dissolved in sesame oil, is also used in some cannabis research. Pilot data on THC by K. R. Muller, MD, demonstrates that it is useful for treating tics and appears safe in the short-term, but additional research is needed.

Advocates for using medicinal marijuana point out that conventional drug treatments can result in serious harmful side effects and are often ineffective. Emmy-award winning talk show host Montel Williams has promoted the issue of legalized medical marijuana. He says marijuana helps his multiple sclerosis symptoms by relieving pain in his legs and feet and controls tremors and spasms better than conventional medications, with fewer side effects.

On the flip side, the National Center on Addiction and Substance Abuse reported in April 2004, that an increasing number of children, at younger ages than ever before, are being treated for marijuana addiction. There is also a reported significant growth in the potency of marijuana over the last 15 years. Studies suggest that in gestation, using marijuana prior to conception is not advisable and may suppress the immune system of the fetus. Cognitive damage among long-term users is also possible. Thus, the potential side effects of marijuana must be recognized.

Dale Gieringer, PhD, on marijuana as medicine

We approached a leader in the fight to legalize medicinal marijuana, Dr. Dale Gieringer, for his insights. He is co-author of the *Medical Marijuana Handbook: A Guide to Therapeutic Use.* He wrote for ACN:

> There has been a tremendous resurgence of interest in medical cannabis research in recent years after passage of medical marijuana laws in California (1996) and in other states. More than 250 indications for medical marijuana have been reported. Many of these conditions are movement-related disorders such as seizures, muscle spasticity, etc. Actual research has been severely stifled by the Drug Enforcement Administration, National Institute on Drug Abuse, and the Federal Drug Administration. However, GW Pharmaceuticals in Wiltshire, United Kingdom, has been proceeding with clinical trials of cannabis extracts for treatment of multiple sclerosis. The California Center for Medicinal Cannabis Research is also looking at marijuana and multiple sclerosis. A number of surveys completed by multiple sclerosis patients indicate that most find marijuana use reduces spasms and pain.
>
> Inhalation is the preferred dosage route for most patients using medical marijuana, because the effects can be immediately gauged and dosage adjusted by self-titration. Patients who use oral preparations typically complain about over and under dosages, as the bioavailability of ingested THC is highly variable and hard to predict. On the other hand, smoking marijuana poses obvious concerns regarding respiratory health. For this reason, there is interest in developing alternative methods of inhalation. One particularly promising technology under investigation is the use of vaporizers that heat marijuana to a temperature where medically active cannabinoids are emitted without combustion and generation of smoke toxins.

Editor: Public opinion polls indicate that more than 70% of Americans support legalizing medical marijuana; many states, as well as Canada, and a growing number of European countries, have already done so. (See *www.norml.org* for updates.) Dale Gieringer's article, above, was written prior to a Supreme Court ruling (June 2005) determining that federal anti-drug laws trump state laws that allow the use of medical marijuana. This means that even those suffering pain from cancer or other serious medical problems can be arrested for using marijuana prescribed by their physician. We will keep readers updated on this issue in our publication, *Latitudes Online* (see page 274).

The role of inflammation and immune function

For decades, doctors who are considered environmental physicians have promoted the concept of "brain allergy," a condition in which the brain is the target organ for an allergic or immune response. The condition was described by William H. Philpott, MD, in *Brain Allergies,* first printed in 1980 and updated in 2000. A practicing psychiatrist before retiring, Dr. Philpott told ACN that he believes many cases of tic disorders are symptomatic of a brain allergy. Many other reports to ACN confirm this. This concept has not traditionally been held by those in conventional medicine; therefore much of our organization's work has involved collecting related data and raising awareness of the importance of the immune system in tic symptoms.

We have been excited that in recent years, scientists have made new discoveries linking the autoimmune/inflammatory process to the development of tic symptoms and the onset of obsessive-compulsive disorder following a *streptococcus* (strep throat) infection. This condition is referred to by the acronym PANDAS (see below). Then, in 2005, James Leckman, MD, and colleagues at Yale University School of Medicine completed research on tics and TS that documents the immune system's inflammatory response and its involvement with tics. The topic of the immune system and tic disorders is discussed in more detail in Section 4.

PANDAS

Several years ago, a form of tic disorder known as *pediatric autoimmune neuropsychiatric disorder associated with group A streptococci* (PANDAS) was identified. Some experts believe that PANDAS, which manifests as an explosive onset of tics, symptoms of obsessive-compulsive disorder (OCD), and/or anxiety, is caused by a strep infection. This comparatively recent PANDAS discovery resulted from groundbreaking work by Susan Swedo, MD, of the National Institute of Mental Health, and her colleagues.

The underlying cause of PANDAS seems similar to the streptococcal infection associated with Sydenham's chorea. In the 1950s, scientists had found that some children developed a movement disorder known as Sydenham's chorea months after having rheumatic fever. (Rheumatic fever is caused by streptococcal infection.)

Research in the field of PANDAS is evolving. The National Institute of Mental Health (2005) recommends that antibiotics not be given as a treatment or preventive measure for PANDAS until further studies have been conducted. However, some reports suggest that treatment with antibiotics, particularly penicillin or a cephalosporin (eg, Keflex, Lorabid), can sometimes improve symptoms of PANDAS and prevent future occurrence, although no definitive therapy has been established. Recent research found that long term use of penicillin and azithromycin reduced neuropsychiatric symptoms in a group of PANDAS subjects. Reports to ACN, though few in number, suggest that many approaches to strengthening the immune system and avoiding triggers that are presented in this book can be of benefit to some diagnosed with PANDAS. (Please read Chapter 18 on the effect of antibiotic use on *Candida albicans* and the need for probiotic therapy when undergoing long-term antibiotic treatments.)

> Recent research (Snider 2005) found that long-term use of penicillin and azithromycin reduced neuropsychiatric symptoms in a group of PANDAS subjects.

Other therapies being explored for PANDAS include *plasmapheresis* for the removal of autoantibodies and intravenous immunoglobulin. Plasmapheresis requires transferring blood out of the body, filtering it to remove autoantibodies, and returning it to the body. This is obviously a major intervention. *Intravenous immunoglobulin* involves administering intravenous immunoglobulin that contains antibodies normally present in adult human blood. This therapy has been used for decades in the treatment of infectious, inflammatory, or autoimmune diseases. It is also used to treat certain autoimmune disorders.

Presently, PANDAS is considered to be a separate category from classic tic disorders or TS (see page 4). Whether this separate status will continue remains to be seen. Dr. Swedo's discovery has opened the door for research into the immune system as an important player in tic symptoms and OCD. This is a relatively new finding, and therefore not all physicians are familiar with PANDAS. If you believe the tic disorder you are encountering might be a result of infection, or if symptoms developed in a dramatic and sudden manner, request that your physician consider this possibility. For more on PANDAS, please see an article on our website (*www.Latitudes.org*) by Dr. Aristo Vojdani. A search for information about PANDAS should also include the website for the National Institute of Mental Health available at *www.nimh.nih.gov*.

Dr. Gerald Erenberg invites proposals

Gerald Erenberg, MD, former chairman for the medical advisory board of the national Tourette Syndrome Association (TSA) and a pediatric neurologist, wrote this message for inclusion in this book.

The treatment of any chronic disorder is unsatisfactory unless the treatment always cures the disorder and never leads to unwanted side effects. Unfortunately, such a magical treatment is not available for TS or for any other medical condition. Currently, the only problem medical science is able to cure is one in which bacterial infections are treated with antibiotics. As we only have imperfect treatments, it is important and natural that all avenues of treatment be explored.

The Tourette Syndrome Association (TSA) is quite aware of the community's interest in alternative therapies, as traditional medical treatment is not curative, does not help everyone, and may lead to adverse side effects. All concerned are hopeful that future scientific research will lead to new and safe ways of treating TS. Just as medical treatment is not helpful for everyone and must be viewed cautiously, the same is true for alternative therapies.

The TSA receives approximately 80 requests for research funds each year. Unfortunately, it is rare for any of the alternative therapies to be studied through the scientific method, though TSA is currently funding a study on the possible benefit of omega-3 oil in the treatment of TS. More studies such as this one would be welcomed. A protocol for submitting research proposals to the TSA to be considered for funding is available on request by sending an e-mail to *ts@tsa-usa.org,* or by calling (718) 224-2999, ext. 222.

Information about all approaches to treating TS is helpful, and I commend Sheila J. Rogers (Director, ACN) for her ongoing efforts to inform the Tourette syndrome community of new ideas.

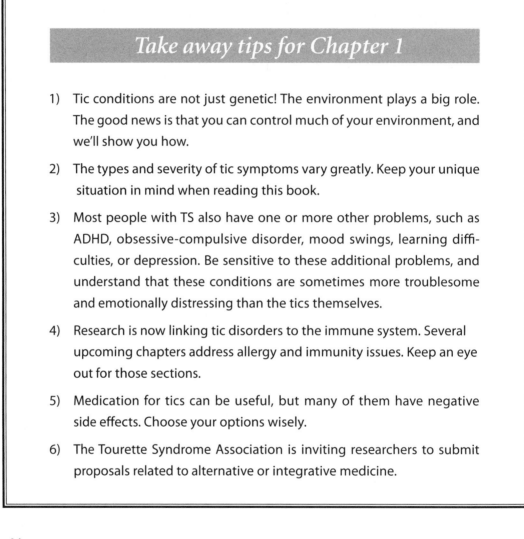

Take away tips for Chapter 1

1) Tic conditions are not just genetic! The environment plays a big role. The good news is that you can control much of your environment, and we'll show you how.

2) The types and severity of tic symptoms vary greatly. Keep your unique situation in mind when reading this book.

3) Most people with TS also have one or more other problems, such as ADHD, obsessive-compulsive disorder, mood swings, learning difficulties, or depression. Be sensitive to these additional problems, and understand that these conditions are sometimes more troublesome and emotionally distressing than the tics themselves.

4) Research is now linking tic disorders to the immune system. Several upcoming chapters address allergy and immunity issues. Keep an eye out for those sections.

5) Medication for tics can be useful, but many of them have negative side effects. Choose your options wisely.

6) The Tourette Syndrome Association is inviting researchers to submit proposals related to alternative or integrative medicine.

Notes:

_____

_____

_____

2

Families Find Nonconventional Answers

WHEN IT COMES TO INVESTIGATING NEW EFFORTS to prevent and reduce tics, parents are often on the front lines. This chapter introduces the accounts of 11 families who investigated and then initiated innovative approaches to tic disorders. Each report summarizes these successful efforts and is representative of other reports received by the Association for Comprehensive NeuroTherapy (ACN) on an ongoing basis. Most of the patients and families in these accounts were dealing with major tic symptoms that had been diagnosed as Tourette syndrome. These cases were selected to emphasize the point that even serious tic disorders can be addressed without medications. The methods and technical terms used in these accounts are discussed in upcoming chapters.

Common themes

The subjects of nutritional deficiency, food sensitivity, infection, and allergy occur in a number of these reports. The percentage of people with tics who find these factors to be connected to symptoms is not yet known, but these subject areas are clearly among the most common in the observations reported to ACN.

Many of the nondrug medical techniques mentioned in the accounts are not truly "alternative." They are standard medical approaches that are not routinely applied to tic disorders. Some of the interventions are also simply commonsense efforts, such as avoiding exposure to toxic chemicals and improving the diet, some of the first steps you might take as you begin to take control of the elements that can affect a tic disorder.

You will see that in most situations, these are not simple quick-fixes. Personal effort at identifying triggers for tics and trying new treatments, alone or in combination, was required. It is also important to bear in mind that people are biologically different. What benefits one person may not benefit another and could even temporarily worsen symptoms until the treatment is adjusted or stopped. There is not a "one size fits all" answer. In some cases, the authors gave permission for their names to be used. Other stories are presented anonymously or with fictitious names.

Keeping case reports in perspective

Positive anecdotal or clinical reports are often criticized as being merely the result of the use of a placebo (the placebo effect). In this scenario, patients expect to get better with a treatment and they do, even when that therapy was a "dummy" or a sugar pill.

Thus, cautious interpretation of anecdotal evidence is justified. However, being overly dismissive of case reports can result in overlooking valid medical insights. We must take care to avoid rejecting reports simply because the treatment is contrary to current thought or because of a narrow and rigid reliance on published studies.

Critics will point out that research literature does not support many of the approaches described in this chapter as potential treatments for tics. Does this mean the techniques are ineffective? No. It simply means they have not been formally studied and that neither positive nor negative findings exist. Clinical or anecdotal reports generally precede studies. Research on many of these efforts will follow, but it may take decades; therefore, you have a choice to make. You can wait for the results of studies to be published, or you can explore new approaches now. The reader is reminded that all treatments in medicine have their benefits and burdens, and these are less defined for newer approaches.

The hope is that accounts such as these will encourage you in your own search for answers and that they will pave the way for future investigation and research.

✥

Nancy and Jim's children

When our first child developed serious tics, my husband and I were stunned. When our second and third sons also began suffering from tics, we were in despair. But let me start at the beginning.

Toby's symptoms began with repeated throat clearing when he was nearly five years old. A few weeks later, I came home from work and found him sitting on the sofa, his arms flailing about and throwing his head back. He made little squeaky bird noises in addition to the throat clearing. I asked him to sit still, but he said he couldn't. He promptly fell off the sofa.

After ruling out epilepsy, the medical specialist advised us that only the drugs that are used for hypertension or psychosis could help Toby's disorder—Tourette syndrome (TS). After hearing the doctor describe a few of the major side effects associated with these medications, I answered that I wanted to try alternative therapies first. After all, Toby was so young. He said I would be wasting my money and would be back for a prescription. Well—we never went back!

Searching for answers

The next few years were difficult. We took Toby to many natural therapy practitioners, and most treatments did not seem to help. Physical adjustments used in chiropractic treatment, however, did stop or slow the tics for seven to ten days after each appointment.

We noticed the tics were worse after Toby watched television or played on a computer, and if Toby went to the cinema, he would tic for days afterward. Aside from this, we had no clue what was causing his problem. The tics were transient and changing, and they seemed to be getting more severe. Then signs of obsessions and compulsions began; he had to touch things the same amount of times with both hands, among other behaviors.

My husband and I went through a roller coaster of emotions. None of the books we had read on tic disorders gave us much hope, and we still wanted to avoid strong medications. But we couldn't find the support in Australia that we needed.

This same year, our second and third sons (Greg and Frankie) also developed tics. Greg's came on without warning. He had explosive vocal tics and also showed obsessive-compulsive tendencies. This distressed him greatly. I used to dread picking him up from school because his behavior was frightening. He would hold these tics in for most of the day, only allowing himself to yell (one of his tics) when playing on the playground so other children would think it was part of a game. Then, as soon as the car door shut he would let the tics out. The intensity of them in a confined space was unbelievable. Once home, there would be tears and rages as he let go of his frustrations. We all bore the brunt of the experience. Eventually we tried home schooling, which took the pressure off as he could tic all day.

When Frankie developed tics they were much milder and involved only his legs.

A major breakthrough

Finally, after three years of struggling to find answers, I came across ACN's website (*www.Latitudes.org*). This was the first time I had found anything to give us hope. I felt total relief and was in tears. Having one child with TS is bad enough, but when the other children showed signs, it was too much for me to handle.

I learned a great deal from the site's forum, where people share their ideas. Much of the discussion was about diet. We had always been food conscious and gave the children simple foods (or so I thought) with lots of water to drink. This is why I didn't suspect a link between what they ate and the tics. Then I heard about salicylates, amines, and natural monosodium glutamate (MSG) (see Chapter 16) in fruits and vegetables. I also learned about the books *Fed Up: Understanding How Food Affects Your Child and What You Can Do About It* and *The Failsafe Cookbook,* both by Sue Dengate, of the Food Intolerance Network, for children with ADHD and related symptoms. For three weeks, we followed Dengate's strict diet that eliminated artificial additives and suspect foods. The results were amazing. Toby's tics decreased by approximately 50%, Greg's rages and mood swings stopped, and he became a calm child with almost no tics! Frankie's leg tics went away altogether.

I was concerned about their nutrient intake on the diet, so we put them on a low-allergy multivitamin, taurine (an amino acid), magnesium phosphate tissue salts (homeopathic), and vitamin C powder. Soon Toby's tics were reduced to almost nothing, and the boys no longer showed obsessive-compulsive behaviors.

Seeing is believing

Who would have dreamed that a diet and supplements would make such a difference? My theory was proven when Toby went on a school-sponsored camp for four nights last year. He was looking forward to it because he was used to sleepovers and got along well with his classmates. Before leaving home, he was 99% tic-free, with even his teacher commenting on how quiet the tics had been. At camp, with its usual outdoor activities, candy was supposedly banned, but I know some was available. The meals included typical camp food: sausages, chips, colored cordial (i.e., Kool Aid), and colored jelly (i.e., Jello), as well as very little plain water.

> Toby had been doing so well that we opted not to send him [to camp] with his special diet, and we withheld his supplements so he could be "normal" for the week. When we picked him up on return, he was a different child. He was very jittery, couldn't stand still, and could barely talk because of his tics.

Toby had been doing so well that we opted not to send him with his special diet, and we withheld his supplements so he could be "normal" for the week. When we picked him up on return, he was a different child. He was very jittery, couldn't stand still, and could barely talk because of his tics. He was throwing his head back, and his arms and legs were flailing about. His teacher, who had gone on the trip, turned to me in tears. She couldn't believe the difference in him.

As soon as we got into the car, Toby burst out crying. He was inconsolable, and by the time we got home he was in a rage and out-of-control. I had to hold him until he calmed down. I put him back on the strict diet and supplements, and after ten days of working to detoxify his body, his health was mostly restored. Now even Toby knows what triggers his tics, and he is more careful with his food intake.

When Toby goes off the diet, or if he becomes sick with a cold or gastrointestinal bug, the tics surface, but when the virus clears up the tics now disappear. He is so much better! As far as I know, there is no genetic TS link in our families, but we do have food intolerances on both sides. I am sure that the symptoms my boys show are greatly due to the combination of artificial colors, preservatives and flavors in foods, as well as salicylates, amines, and natural glutamates. Nutritional deficiencies also needed to be addressed.

I had the boys' blood tested for heavy metals because I was worried about mercury from vaccinations they had received, and because we ate a lot of fish that can contain mercury. All the results were at normal levels, except aluminum, which was "off the scale." (I had been cooking in aluminum pots!) I am now working on reducing the blood levels of aluminum by avoiding exposure and by introducing nutrients, and will have their blood metal levels retested at some point. We have also learned that allergy can play a role, and we are trying to reduce dust and other contaminants in the home.

Matthew

Julia Ross, MA, author of The Diet Cure *and* The Mood Cure, *shared an account of the recovery of a boy named Matthew who had attention deficit hyperactivity disorder (ADHD) and TS. The dietary and nutritional therapy recommended by her clinic was so effective that Matthew was able to accompany Ross to a medical conference to tell his story to the audience. Julia Ross is founder and executive director of Recovery Systems, a California clinic that specializes in treating mood, eating, and addiction problems through counseling, nutrient therapy, and biochemical balancing. Ross is a leader in the field of nutritional psychology.*

Julia Ross:

Matthew had experienced symptoms of ADHD for years. Though he was a challenge to teachers in his private elementary school, the problems were manageable. Then one fall, everything seemed to break loose. Behavior and hyperactivity symptoms worsened, and tics developed—including swearing and other vocal tics. The school staff could no longer maintain Matthew in the classroom and began pushing for the family to see a psychiatrist for medications.

Matthew's mother was committed to natural health approaches. Matthew's dad, a conventional businessman, was at least open to new treatment ideas. On the first visit to our clinic, their nine-year-old son was tearing through the clinic counseling office, running here and there. When he settled down long enough for us to talk, I realized Matthew was bright enough to understand that his problems might worsen and stay with him for the rest of his life. He was willing to try our recommendations. After all, he didn't like the tics, and he didn't enjoy getting in trouble at school.

Nutritional therapy begins

Based on history, laboratory test results, and other presenting symptoms—including chronic digestive and respiratory problems—a gluten- and dairy-free diet was recommended. Matthew and his family were also instructed to avoid sweets, artificial colors and flavors, and preservatives. We advised them to include protein in Matthew's diet three times a day. Matthew wasn't happy to give up some of his favorite foods, but he agreed to give things a try to see what would happen.

Other recommendations included introducing select nutrients: a multivitamin with minerals, omega-3 caplets, pycnogenol (an antioxidant) to help his focus and concentration, and GABA (gamma amino butyric acid) with tyrosine (an amino acid). He was also given St. John's wort glycerin tincture to help normalize serotonin levels because he could not swallow the recommended tryptophan capsules, nor could he tolerate the taste of the powder that his mother emptied out of the capsules, even when it was mixed with juice. Within a few weeks, Matthew was doing much better. After one month, the family reported that tics and hyperactivity seemed something of the past.

When they came back to the clinic for a follow-up, his mother explained that Matthew was about to have a birthday and wanted to go off the diet for the weekend. This was agreed to, and he had pizza and other treats. To Matthew's surprise, his behavioral and tic symptoms immediately came back with a vengeance. From then on, Matthew stopped begging for foods that were off his diet—in this case, milk in the pizza's cheese and gluten in the wheat crust, and, of course, sugary birthday party foods.

Follow-up with Matthew

I followed up with Matthew when he was 13 years old—five years after our first meeting. He had maintained all of his improvements. He told me he had been able to stop most of the supplements, but he was still following the restricted diet. He admitted that one of the hardest things to deal with was when kids teased him because he wasn't eating the same foods they were having. But, he added, "They don't tease me nearly as much as they did when I had the tics and behavior problems!"

✦

Valerie and Marty

I live in Midwest America with my husband and two children. Our daughter, Valerie is 16 years old, our son is 11. Other than testing positive for allergies when she was three years of age, Valerie was always a healthy, bright, and athletic girl. In 1991, when she was five years old, she began to display tic symptoms. It wasn't until 1995 that we took her to our family physician; the symptoms had worsened and were now uncontrollable. The physician told us these were transient tics that would only last about one year. I was unsure of his diagnosis and wanted a second opinion, as her tics were now both motor (movement) and vocal. They were also increasing in intensity.

The next year, she was diagnosed with TS and ADHD. She was put on standard medication. We saw no improvement, only negative side effects. Over time, we consulted several physicians, and many medications were prescribed.

Making the allergy connection

I finally found a physician who specialized in TS. She seemed very knowledgeable and straightforward. I learned about the Tourette Syndrome Association and took Valerie to a Tourette summer camp. There, I noted that many children used asthma inhalers, my daughter being one of them. I thought that to be odd. Was it just coincidental?

Our son Marty was born in 1992. He was chronically ill, always in and out of the hospital and undergoing surgery for various reasons. When he was three months old, his physician prescribed a bronchodilator medication used for asthmatics. He also received adrenal corticosteroids and breathing machine treatments. He was about six years old when we first noticed he was having tics. In the meantime, I was searching the Internet for information about asthma and tics.

My son was bright, and so he qualified for the gifted program at school. His tic symptoms, however, were now bad enough that they needed to be treated. Yet, he was already on several medications for his asthma, and I didn't want to put him on any more drugs.

When he turned eight years old, I scheduled an appointment with the same Tourette specialist my daughter was seeing and continued collecting information day and night, looking for a better solution.

I felt that a new allergist would be of great benefit. Marty and I hoped we could decrease the number of medications he had to take. I searched and found *www.Latitudes.org*, the website for ACN and *Latitudes* magazine. After reading the information on the site, I realized that the many children with inhalers at the camp probably had allergies, and the connection with tics was not just a coincidence. The next morning I called to cancel my son's doctor appointment. I told the physician that I was going to see an environmental physician (see Section 4) instead. Her reply was, "Well, if you choose to take that route. . . ."

> After reading the information on the website (*www.Latitudes.org*), I realized that the many children with inhalers at the camp probably had allergies, and the connection with tics was not just a coincidence.

I jumped in and said, "Who wouldn't! Why would you want to give medications for something my kids don't have? We do not have a history of Tourette syndrome in our family, but we do have allergies."

At this point the doctor said, "I have the name of a website you should visit." I was quite surprised when she gave me the *www.Latitudes.org* site. I told her I'd already been there, and angrily asked why I was not told of this all the years I had been going to that clinic. (If you only knew the suffering my daughter went through at school when peers and teachers kept telling her to stop making faces when they knew she couldn't help it!)

Finding their way to restored health

I took both of the children to see an environmental medicine specialist, James W. Willoughby, DO, in Liberty, Missouri. (Over time, this doctor's treatment has made an incredible difference in controlling our children's symptoms.) We learned that they both had chemical intolerances and that my son had food intolerances that affected the tics. My daughter had food sensitivities and could not tolerate perfumes. Watching what environmental elements my children were exposed to and what they ate resulted in a significant improvement in their health.

Valerie is almost completely off the prescribed medications that she took for many years. My son has gone from a regimen of eight daily asthma medications to just one. He was also diagnosed with Candidiasis, a yeast overgrowth, for which he was treated.

I limit or rotate foods to which they are sensitive so they don't consume great amounts of any of them. I can sense how much of one food my son can have before he is on "overload." For example, if he eats too much corn, it will trigger a major tic. The allergy treatment we used greatly improved my son's overall health and school attendance. Valerie's allergic tics, on the other hand, are more affected by chemicals than by foods.

I love to share our story with everyone I can, and I hope it helps others.

Aaron

Cheri Marshall of Orlando, Florida wrote this account about her son, Aaron:

Specialists diagnosed mild attention deficit disorder (ADD) without hyperactivity in my son when he was in kindergarten, during which time he also began wearing glasses. The pediatric ophthalmologist noticed his eye-rolling but didn't feel it was serious. We now know that this was probably his first tic.

Aaron did very well at school and everything else he attempted until fourth grade, when attention difficulties seemed to intensify. We resisted attempts by the school to push us into a Ritalin course of treatment, especially as his physician felt it was unnecessary. Aaron has always been a delightful child with many talents and a wonderful sense of humor. However, in December 1999, a few weeks after he turned 10 years old, he became deeply depressed, afraid, and paranoid. It was distressing for the whole family.

Major tics begin

Within a few weeks, Aaron started manifesting major tics—banging his chin and a whiplash motion of his head and neck, along with many loud vocal tics. Obsessive-compulsive symptoms were also intense.

We took him to see a developmental pediatrician who said we were seeing the onset of Tourette's in Aaron. He also gave me literature on OCD, as he felt that Aaron was showing a common blend of tics and compulsions. He advised us to stay away from medications unless it became absolutely necessary.

As we researched TS and OCD, my husband realized that the "bad habits" he had been accused of having as a child were probably also tics and OCD, and he recalled that his father had similar symptoms. We had always just labeled his father's strange noises and actions as eccentric. Now we believed our family had a hereditary link to these disorders.

Teachers at Aaron's school were insisting on his being medicated. An ultimatum was finally issued: medicate or withdraw. We transferred Aaron to a private school for kids with learning disabilities and other special needs. Nearly one year after TS and OCD were diagnosed in Aaron, we began seeing a psychologist to help Aaron with the despondency and difficulties he was experiencing. Once a happy-go-lucky child with lots of friends, he was now hiding from people because he was different, ticcing uncontrollably, and suffering debilitating obsessions, compulsions, anxieties, and depression.

The psychologist told us we were "denying Aaron a full quality of life" by not putting him on medications and dismissed our concerns about potential side effects. Aaron also began to tell us we were unfair to withhold medications that could make him better. We began to feel guilty for not medicating him and took him to a neurologist who reinforced this message. Reluctantly we agreed to administer a standard TS medication on which both physicians agreed.

So started a downward spiral and a nightmare journey of life on brain drugs.

Frightening reactions to medication

Within one month of starting drug treatment, Aaron became psychotic, and his tics and OCD became worse. When I reported this, the doctors said he should see a psychiatrist as he obviously needed a pharmaceutical combination. While waiting for our first consultation, Aaron developed a severe tic that was so intense he had to be hospitalized. It was a horrifying time, especially because the hospital psychiatrist wanted to admit him to the "psych ward" for disturbed kids! I flatly refused and stayed by his bedside all that week. They pumped Aaron full of enough intravenous drugs to sedate him and released him into my care on the condition that I add an antidepressant to the tic medication.

I'll cut a long story short by saying that we endured one year of watching Aaron suffer adverse side effects from various medications that were far worse than his TS symptoms had ever been. We were truly alarmed at the severity and intensity of his tics while on medications; they were often totally disabling and sometimes very scary. His grades plummeted, and his love for music and artistic expression waned. He no longer had any energy, motivation, or inspiration.

The physicians responded to this downturn by adding more medications, which we now understand were just worsening things. Finally they tried him on yet another drug.

Aaron nearly died from his severe reaction to the drug; he then began exhibiting tardive dyskinesia, a different and serious movement disorder that is a known side effect of one of the medications! We all realized this madness had to end. Aaron begged us to take him off the medications, and we willingly agreed. By the way, the condition PANDAS (see pages 13–15) had been ruled out in his case.

Welcoming Aaron back

We enlisted the help of an open-minded and compassionate psychiatrist who helped withdraw Aaron from the medications—another horrid experience. In spite of dire warnings from his former physicians, as soon as the withdrawal period was over, we immediately started to see improvement in his condition.

Thanksgiving that year (2001) was a special time as we began to see glimmers of the "old" Aaron and his wonderful personality, not the overweight, despondent, and disturbed zombie that he had been the previous year. We were truly grateful.

I home schooled him for the rest of that school year while his body healed and he recovered. I researched and we began to explore alternative treatments, as I realized I would have to investigate the possibilities myself. We found integrative physicians and were referred to a therapist who started Aaron on acupuncture, biofeedback treatment, and homeopathic remedies. We were delighted to see immediate and remarkable improvement!

> We found integrative physicians and were referred to a therapist who started Aaron on acupuncture, biofeedback treatment, and homeopathic remedies. We were delighted to start seeing immediate and remarkable improvement.

At this time, I learned about new ideas for nutritional support, and my holistic team helped formulate a comprehensive treatment protocol for Aaron. His obsession and compulsions all but vanished, his tics soon became mild, and his attention difficulties were lessened. We also dealt with *Candida albicans* yeast in his system (see Chapter 18) and slowly detoxified him from elevated mercury levels.

In addition to agreeing to take supplements, Aaron willingly adopted a healthful diet and began avoiding artificial foods, especially colorings and NutraSweet/aspartame type sweeteners, monosodium glutamate, and other additives. We stopped using pesticides, strong household cleaning chemicals, and perfumes, as these triggered his tics. Also, we began eliminating dust mites and mold exposure as much as we could.

I have tried to make these modifications without being fanatical. It has been interesting to see how, even at 15 years of age, Aaron has chosen to self-regulate his intake and exposure to things that can make his symptoms worse.

Sharing with others

So, where is Aaron now in this journey? Well, he is doing wonderfully! He has gone from bringing home failing grades during that year on medications to all "A"s and "B"s. He has been able to fully integrate back into the school system and is happy at his high school. He was awarded a countywide public school "Local Hero" award for an essay/speech he wrote that explains what it is like to live with TS and to overcome the challenges it presents. He has developed his musical skills and is busily engaged in faith-related volunteer projects to help others.

Aaron is upfront in telling people about his condition and is determined to educate people in that regard. I am thrilled to see how my son has met the challenge that so dramatically changed his life and devastated our family.

Jonathan

Jonathan began showing signs of eye-blinking when he was six years old. I didn't think much of it but took him to our pediatrician who assured us it was a common transient tic that would probably go away. Sure enough, the tics lessened but later resurfaced. We basically ignored them until, at nine years of age, a vocal tic began—similar to a hiccup—with a soft gasp.

Although not especially noticeable, the new tic was a red flag. I headed back to the pediatrician and left his office with a referral for a neurologist in hand. Meanwhile, we went on vacation, and the tics became more severe. Tics now occurred up to 40 times per minute, and the vocal tics were very loud. Frantic, we called the emergency department and were told there was nothing that could be done. It was an awful experience.

On returning home, we consulted with two neurologists. They both diagnosed Jonathan's symptoms as TS, and, again, we were told that there was nothing we could do at this point. "It might get better in several years, but then again it might not." We were told that if it became worse, we could return to talk about drug therapy.

I was so frustrated! Was I expected to just sit around and do nothing? I headed for the computer and began to do research. I subscribed to *Latitudes,* and it gave me hope. My husband and I began to educate ourselves on wellness issues.

Treatment at The Optimal Wellness Center

A few months later, I learned of Dr. Joseph Mercola, DO, founder and director of the The Optimal Wellness Center in Schaumburg, Illinois. I met with Dr. Mercola, as well as a nutritionist and an osteopathic physician at his center. Jonathan had seasonal sinus allergies, and Dr. Mercola recommended a diet that excluded dairy products. Jonathan had been drinking about four glasses of milk a day since he was one year old! Soon the tics were greatly reduced. Junk food was then eliminated—we avoided artificial flavors and colors and cut way back on sugar-laden foods. We learned by trial and error how these items affected Jonathan's tics. I also reduced his grain intake. Our family is Asian, and we ate rice almost every day, plus Jonathan loved pasta. I switched to organic foods as much as possible and now realize how important it was to change that aspect of his diet.

In books by Doris Rapp, MD, I learned of natural products that can be used in the home, and we then changed our cleaning, laundry, and personal products to avoid toxic exposure. Tics had now subsided to the point of being mild, if occurring at all. Jonathan received osteopathic manipulative treatment and craniosacral therapy at the Optimal Wellness Center. After each treatment, his sinus allergies were better. Other aspects of treatment included homeopathic medicine to assist his body in detoxification; supplements, including essential fatty acids, and vitamin C; and acidophilus to restore balance to his gastrointestinal tract.

> Jonathan's tics are so well under control now that no one would believe the ordeal with which we had to deal. His body is less reactive, and he does not have to follow the dietary restrictions quite as strictly as before.

Jonathan's tics are so well under control now that no one would believe the ordeal we had been through. His body is less reactive, and he does not have to follow the dietary restrictions quite as strictly as before. I know many families start their young children on strong drugs because they don't know to try alternatives before resorting to medications. I hope our story will help them realize that there are options they can consider. We feel very fortunate.

✥

Maria

I have struggled with Tourette syndrome throughout my life. Therefore, I was heart-broken when my six-year-old daughter, Maria, first showed signs of the disorder. She then began having more frequent facial tics and also made little noises. I knew too well the challenges that could lie ahead for her. She's such a good sport and so well-behaved; it was killing me to watch this happen to her. My wife and I didn't emphasize the motor (movement) and vocal tics, so fortunately Maria was not self-conscious about them.

I had tried standard medications myself and decided I was better off without them. I certainly didn't want my little girl on these drugs, so I started searching for answers, beginning the investigative journey. After a phone call to Sheila J. Rogers, director of ACN, I decided to locate an environmental physician to find out whether allergies, diet, and/or environment were possibly playing a role. I knew my own tics improved when I gave up alcohol, so I was open to the concept that dietary factors could make a difference.

Our first visit to an environmental physician

Without mentioning the tics, I told Maria that I wanted to find out if she had allergies. I dragged her and my skeptical wife to the office of Joseph S. Wojcik, MD, in Bronxville, New York. I will never forget what happened at the clinic! In fact, if I had not seen it with my own eyes, I wouldn't have believed it possible.

Maria received intradermal skin testing (not the "scratch" test) to determine the items to which she might have allergies. She had no idea what she was being tested for, nor the real purpose in her being there. When they tested the first few substances, there was no reaction that I could see, though the nurse noticed a change in skin reaction, on which the treatment is primarily based. Then they tested her for mold, dust, cat dander, and different foods. Her personality began to take on big changes. Although previously sitting calmly and quietly, Maria now began moving around, and tics began to surface. Then her body began jerking, and she made noises. Her comments became silly and inappropriate, and she was repeating words in a high-pitched voice. She was hyperactive and talking incessantly to office staff to the point of being inappropriate. It was very out of character for her. My wife and I sat there with our mouths open! We were greatly relieved when neutralizing doses "brought her back."

Maria was given an allergy treatment vial prepared specifically for her sensitivities and later received her first neutralizing dose. As I looked at her later that evening, I realized that her little body was the calmest I had seen in it months.

Making adjustments with positive results

It has been two years since first visiting Dr. Wojcik, and Maria is doing very well. We have made dietary changes at home and observe that when we are lax with the diet, especially with sweets, minor tics creep in, and we have to tighten things up again. After learning that she is allergic to cats, we found someone to take our cat. We now see a pattern that when she visits a friend's house and plays with a cat, she returns home making unusual verbal noises. Otherwise, the noises do not occur. We were planning to move and made it a point to locate a mold-free home. Maria had tested allergic to mold, and our previous home, where her tics had been the most extreme, contained a lot of mold.

Maria receives allergy injections a couple of times a week, and we occasionally return to Dr. Wojcik for a fine-tuning of her treatment plan. It is such a relief to know that we have some control over this condition. As a father, that means the world to me. The changes we made have also helped my own symptoms.

✦

Griff

This is a description, as told to the author, of the experience of Griffin Wakem and his mother, Ginger, to whom this book is dedicated:

In 1986, Ginger Wakem and her husband were desperately dealing with their son's Tourette syndrome (TS) symptoms. Griffin (Griff) had developed normally and was clearly bright. He seemed healthy, but when he was six years old, he developed some mild tics. By the fourth grade, something had gone terribly wrong. His mother recalls, "Griff disrupted his gifted classes with ear-splitting shrieks. He made noises, kicked desks, and waved his arms. He involuntarily beat his chest so hard with both fists that he damaged the lining of his lungs." After a trip to the emergency department one night, his parents began taping a foam pad to his T-shirt to cushion his chest.

"For six weeks," Ginger said, "the tics were so bad that Griff couldn't even hold a pencil. He was depressed and wished he were dead. And all this was while he was on medication." Students taunted Griff, and at home the family struggled to deal with temper tantrums and mood swings. Tourette's had snatched Ginger and Peter Wakem's talented, sweet-natured boy and given them a nightmare in return.

Positive results at last

After taking Griff to different neurologists and to a psychiatrist, Ginger went into therapy herself to deal with the stress. The following year, a friend recommended that she take her son to an environmental physician. Griff was seen by two environmental physicians in Florida, both of whom were helpful: Kenneth Krischer, MD, in Plantation (recently deceased) and Albert F. Robbins, DO, in Deerfield Beach.

To the family's amazement, Griff was found during testing to have an allergic reaction to corn, egg, and milk—each of which caused different tic symptoms. More testing showed that beet and cane sugar could bring on shrieks, aggressive behavior, and loss of concentration. His eyes itched in response to the introduction of wheat, he sneezed as a reaction to chicken, and he was unable to hold a pencil when tested for tomato. Apple and chocolate brought on some of the worst tics. Griff was also hypersensitive to certain dusts, molds, pollens, and chemicals. Laboratory work revealed nutritional imbalances. The highly reactive state that Griff exhibited is considered unusual and has been referred to as "exquisite sensitivity."

> His eyes itched in response to the introduction of wheat, he sneezed as a reaction to chicken, and he was unable to hold a pencil when tested for tomato.

Standard medications had failed and the family was anxious to help Griff. So, jumping in with both feet, they vigorously removed chemicals and allergens from their home and adjusted Griff's diet. Drug therapy was discontinued, while nutrient and allergy therapy began. Within a few months, the major tics had subsided. Griff's health improved, his grades improved, and "he was a joy to be with once more."

Mom turns advocate

Ginger gradually observed that whenever Griff was inadvertently exposed to something he was allergic or sensitive to, symptoms would flare, though never to the previous degree. "This is a remarkable connection," she thought.

Seeking to help other families, Ginger began collecting and sharing letters she received about similar experiences with twitches and tics. This effort eventually grew into the current Association for Comprehensive NeuroTherapy, now directed by the author of this book, Sheila J. Rogers.

Griff's success story was included in a BBC documentary on TS for the Discovery Health Channel's "Medical Mysteries" series, which has aired several times. Now a successful businessman, Griff agreed to the use of his story and name in the hope that others might be spared the pain that he and his family endured before they learned that allergens and chemical exposures were responsible for his central nervous system problems.

✦

Rami

We are a family with five children living in Israel. Our third son, Rami, was born in 1991 and his symptoms were diagnosed as Tourette syndrome at seven years of age. The pregnancy with Rami occurred during the first Gulf War and was therefore highly stressful. We had Iraqi scuds falling on our heads (our house was literally in the fire zone). In addition, I was in the army and out of the house for long periods.

Rami was hyper from birth. Around six months of age, he seemed increasingly restless and developed severe atopic dermatitis (eczema). After turning two years old, it was clear that Rami needed allergy therapy. Although he did not have attention problems, he became increasingly energetic. His nickname was "the energizer," named after the "Energizer bunny" commercials. He was athletic but required constant attention and direction. We would send Rami on "missions" to run around the block as fast as he could. (We lived in a kibbutz and the war was over, so there was no safety problem). I would time him and send him again and again!

At about four years of age, he began having rage attacks that we did not know how to interpret. He also became overly social and would make immediate physical and social contact with anyone, including strangers. A year later, he was diagnosed only as *not* having attention deficit/hyperactivity disorder. No one had an answer for what he *did* have.

The situation worsened. His rage attacks increased, and he developed obsessions—an abnormal degree of focus on certain themes. As these problems coupled with greater physical power, he began to dominate our lives. It was not long before life seemed almost unbearable. Rami took up skiing, skateboarding, cycling, and karate with success. But during all of this time he had terrible rage attacks, skin allergy and itching, and displayed hyper social behavior.

Rami's negative reaction to Haldol

Around seven years of age, tics burst forth violently. These included head and shoulder jerks. These tics did not disturb him as much as his eye-rolling, which caused concentration problems during reading and sports activities. A nurse arranged an emergency visit to a child neurologist. The neurologist immediately diagnosed his symptoms as TS and prescribed Haldol.

The reaction to Haldol was immediate: the tics subsided by 95%, but his energy was drained. Within days his mental capability and alertness dropped by half, and academic performance slid. We lost our kid and got a zombie instead.

After some weeks, Rami developed a severe school phobia. He would resist going to school and once there, would run away from class and hide, or even run away from school. When trying to perform a physical activity, he would give up after a short time. In addition, his personality began fluctuating. He would be zoned out in school but hyper in the evening, with accompanying rage attacks. When we forgot to administer his Haldol, tics returned within one day and rages and hyperactivity increased. In summary, the Haldol solved the tic problem and dampened the rage temporarily, but it changed his personality entirely, by 180 degrees. We decided the medication was unacceptable.

Our search for an alternative

We tried some behavioral techniques with unclear results. We tried psychological therapy which had negative effects because Rami was resistant. Then we researched options on the Internet and found an alternative therapy that uses fish oil.

About eight months after starting Haldol, I began to gradually substitute fish oil for the drug. Based on advice from other parents on Internet forums, I learned that the introduction of fish oil had to be done carefully and slowly because of the risk of synergistic effects of the medication and the fish oil. In other words, the fish oil could make the Haldol more "effective." I kept a detailed diary and noted any changes in dosages.

I began with giving a capful of fish oil, which contains omega-3 fatty acids, together with the Haldol. After just a few days, I started seeing increased side effects of Haldol. There was more fatigue and zombiness. So I reduced the Haldol by 20%. The side effects subsided slightly. No tics! No rage! Then I doubled the dose of fish oil. Again, the zombiness increased, so I reduced the Haldol by another 20%. This process continued over three months, and the situation finally improved. After five gradual steps like these, we reached a level where we could reduce the Haldol to zero!

What a great day this was. I will never forget it. We were vacationing on a beach on Lake Galilee. Rami was having such a great time that I decided to take the risk and eliminate the medication completely. And voila! Nothing adverse happened. We had weaned him off the medication with no resulting tics, and there was no rage. We got our boy back with his old personality, only improved.

During this time we noticed that his allergy symptoms were reduced, and his need for corticosteroid medication and antihistamines was reduced. Since then (he is now 13 years old) we have learned a lot about nutrition and health. We switched to a high protein, high fat, low carbohydrate diet, and have reduced grain foods. I can say that all of our family is now very healthy.

Has Rami been "cured?"

The answer is no. The same deficiency, which I believe is mainly an enzymatic deficiency in his fatty acid metabolic pathways, still exists. He is being treated with an aggressive diet of fish oil that has to be maintained at a certain ratio of omega-3 to body mass. This means we have to increase his dose gradually as he grows. If we reduce his dose of fish oil or neglect to adjust it to his growing body mass, the negative symptoms return.

Failure to take the fish oil, even for one day, shows in his behavior and rage. Now that he is more mature, he can even describe this feeling of rage. It is very similar to the old rage he used to have: a rapid escalation with shouting and screaming for no apparent reason and then a rapid cool down. We also see that his atopic dermatitis and occasional asthma symptoms respond positively to the correct dosage of fish oil. We have recently started to add other nutrients to his daily protocol as well.

This year our son had his bar mitzvah, six years after receiving a diagnosis of TS. Socially, he is very successful. He has many friends and girls want to be near him. In school he is doing well, not excellent but not badly either. He excels in sports. He is very responsible and warm-hearted—a good boy!

✦

Lisa

In 1997, at age four, our daughter, Lisa, started exhibiting strange movements and behaviors—a head toss and an arm jerk—and she would repeat or say words that were out of context. She also exhibited signs of OCD, manifested as an obsession with hand-washing and a constant need for "just right" behaviors. We were asked to do and say things over and over until they seemed "right" to her. She also experienced wild mood swings—often within minutes.

I researched alternative therapies and met with an environmental physician who is also a psychiatrist in Saratoga, California. He was concerned about Lisa's lifelong constipation, sometimes making only one stool per week. He ordered tests, including a food allergy profile, organic acid urinalysis, stool examination, and a cellular nutrient levels evaluation. Results showed a severe deficiency in calcium, magnesium, zinc, and a few antioxidants. The test also revealed sensitivity to wheat and other gluten grains, numerous other foods, and poor pancreatic enzyme output.

> Results showed a severe deficiency in calcium, magnesium, zinc, and a few antioxidants. The test also revealed sensitivity to wheat and other gluten grains.

Dietary changes, biofeedback, and homeopathy

Lisa's diet was changed to eliminate all gluten and we began to rotate foods. We dropped dairy products from cows, and she was placed on digestive enzymes and a daily drink that included probiotics, glutamine, and other gut-healing supplements. (Probiotics are used to counteract the well-known bacterial imbalance that antibiotics create in the digestive tract; glutamine is an amino acid.) Initially she also took a large amount of vitamin C daily. She gradually improved, and nine months after beginning the gluten-free diet and treatments, she started having completely normal bowel movements every day. Vitamin C was then reduced.

We were referred to a dietician who worked with our other practitioners to develop a nutritional plan, which we carefully followed. Soon Lisa's motor tics disappeared, and they have not returned. We also pursued EEG (electroencephalogram) biofeedback, which seemed to help her moods, and homeopathic treatment with Ananda Zaren in Santa Barbara, California, to address allergies and OCD. Today, the number of food allergies she reacts to have been reduced from 34 to 4, and she only takes supplements and her homeopathic remedy.

Lisa is now ten years old and we are extremely pleased with her progress. It has required a great deal of culinary creativity and a tremendous amount of cooperation on our daughter's part, but Lisa sees how much better she feels when she stays with the program, eats right, and takes her supplements.

✦

Michael

This account was written by Shelly A. Schneider, a freelance writer in St. Louis, Missouri:

Michael began displaying a vocal tic in summer 2000, before first grade. We took our son to his pediatrician, believing he had allergies. We tried Claritin and other over-the-counter products, but nothing seemed to help.

After one month, I decided Michael had simply developed a habit and couldn't function without making grunting type noises—which were by now louder and more frequent. These vocal tics drove me bananas, but the more I needled him to stop, the more he made them. I took him back to his pediatrician, completely frustrated. She completed a physical examination of Michael and declared that his system was "clear."

"Is there anything else you think it could be?" she asked me.

"Could it be Tourette's?" I offered.

Don't ask me how I knew to ask that question. The only thing I knew of TS, I learned from watching an episode of "LA Law" on television! The pediatrician agreed with my thoughts, and gave me the name of a pediatric neurologist in St. Louis. My husband and I took Michael to the specialist. We all noticed his motor tics: pointing his arms straight down, making fists, and gently knocking his fists against his legs, straight-armed fashion. The doctor said that at the very least, Michael had a tic disorder, and he recommended a standard TS drug. I knew enough about this medication to know that I was not about to put my six-year-old son on it.

Finding the help we needed

This is where determination and research skills come into the picture. I am a journalist by training and was relentless in my resolve to relieve my middle child's suffering.

Through 50 hours of research, I came across the name of Tipu Sultan, MD, an environmental allergist in Florissant, Missouri. I called immediately and scheduled an appointment. The paperwork was, quite frankly, a giant pain, but it made me think about Michael, his symptoms, when they began, and how severe they were.

On meeting with Dr. Sultan, we learned that Michael suffered from a number of allergies, and we agreed that his tics were related somewhat to these. St. Louis is known for its airborne allergens and is consistently on the list as one of the top places to avoid if you have allergies.

Tics brought under control

We talked with Michael's teachers about the possibility of placing him in an alternative classroom because his grunting noises were very loud, and he made them every two to three seconds. Per Dr. Sultan, I began giving Michael three desensitization shots per week, and decided to remove dairy products from his diet. He also began taking magnesium supplements. The tics were drastically reduced. You can imagine how happy this made his teacher, his guidance counselor, his classmates, and his family!

> Per Dr. Sultan, I began giving Michael three desensitization shots per week, and decided to remove dairy products from his diet. He was also started on magnesium supplements. The tics were drastically reduced.

Five years later, Michael is still off dairy products, although we do allow some cheese and yogurt once a week or so. Fortunately Michael does not like sweets, though he indulges occasionally. The tics are not really noticeable anymore. In fact, if you didn't know Michael had TS, you might think he just has a cold or simple allergies. His tics include softly clearing his throat and opening and closing his mouth as if his ears are plugged and he's trying to "pop" them. This still comes and goes. He has attention deficit disorder, but like his tics, that is now mild. Socially, Michael has a harder time than our other children, but he is a very loving and caring little boy and really enjoys school. His hobbies include computer games, basketball, and playing with our dog, Fritz. (He wasn't allergic to dogs, thank goodness!)

I cannot imagine having to watch my son on personality-altering and mind-dulling drugs. He is one of the absolute joys in my life, and I thank God each day for Michael. I thank Him, too, for Michael's Tourette's. This neurologic disorder has taught the entire family about patience. We've also learned not to accept as gospel every word from a physician's mouth. We realize how lucky we are. We know children whose symptoms are much more severe than Michael's. My husband and I are very grateful to Dr. Sultan and his staff. We have successful control of Michael's symptoms and are hopeful that they will subside further by the time he enters his high school years. We are truly blessed and hope to give back in any way we can.

A comment on Michael from Tipu Sultan, MD

This child was six years old when first seen with multiple tics consisting of grunting, jerking head backwards, and flapping of hands against his thighs, which had started one year before. The symptoms had been getting progressively worse. Additional symptoms included a short attention span and hay fever beginning in fall 1999, and then again in spring 2000.

His diagnosis included allergic rhinitis because of a runny or stuffy nose, dark circles under his eyes, hay fever, and symptoms of Candidiasis as a result of being given a considerable number of antibiotics in the past.

Skin testing revealed sensitivity to house dust, house dust mites, multiple molds, and spring and fall pollens. Skin testing also confirmed sensitivity to *Candida albicans*. Michael was given desensitization therapy for dust, mold and *Candida albicans*. Nystatin was prescribed as an antifungal (antiyeast) medication. In addition, he was given a multivitamin and minerals in the form of Super Nu-Thera (manufactured by Kirkman, Lake Osewgo, Oregon) as well as essential fatty acid supplements.

Michael had a history of tics becoming progressively worse during the spring and fall pollen seasons, but with immunotherapy, nystatin, and the other treatments mentioned above, his tics have improved considerably during those periods and his respiratory symptoms have also. Mother reported the improvement as falling between 75% and 90%.

✤

Tim

Tim was ten years old when I took him to an osteopathic physician who specializes in manipulative treatment. Tim stood self-consciously in the middle of the examining room as I sat anxiously nearby. Dr. Richard MacDonald (of Palm Beach Gardens, Florida), began:

"What's the problem?"

"My son has Tourette syndrome."

"No, that's not what I asked you. That's just the label he has been given. I asked what the problem is."

"Oh. Well—he has a lot of tics, and they're getting much worse," I said, trying to control my emotions. We were dealing with many facial, neck, shoulder, and eye tics, along with mild vocalizations (little sounds he couldn't help making), compulsions, obsessions, and mood swings.

He replied, "You need to understand that tics are the body's way of letting you know that something is wrong. They are a symptom. They're saying, 'Something is wrong inside—won't you fix it?' The label isn't important."

Hope emerged for the first time.

Recalling one year before

More than a year before this, we had been in the office of a neurologist who specialized in tic disorders. I had assured my son that this man was an expert, and he would help us. After a brief discussion while watching Tim's facial contortions, the doctor said, "You have Tourette syndrome. I can't tell you why you have it, and there is no cure." He looked at me, "He should tell his friends, and you should tell his teachers that this is the way he is. If they care about him, they will accept him. I'd say his tics are a four on a scale of ten.

There's no way of knowing whether they will get better or worse. Go back home, and if the tics get worse during the coming months, you can come back for medication. We don't like to use the drugs unless we must because of their troublesome side effects."

"But isn't there something I can do?" I pleaded.

"No. Just try to avoid stress. The good news is, no one ever died from Tourette syndrome."

I was dismayed and glanced over at Tim, whose blue eyes had filled with tears. After paying the bill we headed for the car, and with each step I grew more indignant and angry. How could a doctor say such discouraging, unhelpful things—and in front of my child! This was "expert" advice?

As I started up the engine I firmly told Tim to forget everything he had just heard, adding, "Don't worry. I'm going to get you some help."

How would I find this help? I had absolutely no idea, but I would not accept that a delightful and previously normal child was being subjected to the ravages of Tourette's without a fight.

A new way of looking at symptoms

Dr. MacDonald, who had suggested that tics were symptoms waiting to be "fixed," promised us he would stay with our case as we looked for answers. Tim received a few craniosacral therapy treatments from him, enough to assure that any structural stressors affecting the condition had been addressed. Meanwhile, Dr. MacDonald helped us locate an environmental physician and allergist, Albert F. Robbins, DO, who hopefully would help us investigate what was causing the tics.

When I took my son to see Dr. Robbins, I had no idea what to expect. Although I didn't think of Tim as allergic, I didn't know where else to turn. He reviewed an environmental history questionnaire that we had filled out in advance. Blood work was done, and Tim was tested for foods he frequently ate. Reaction to dusts, molds, and pollens were also assessed. I was told that many people with tics have chemical sensitivities. Therefore, we were advised to eliminate scented items at home and to stop using toxic cleaners. The idea of Tim having chemical sensitivities seemed a bit far fetched (I'd never heard of this concept before). I nodded my head in agreement but mentally dismissed this advice.

Tim went through several hours of testing over three days, and we received three treatment vials for allergy injections to cover molds, inhalants (dusts and pollens), and foods. At first I found a nurse in the neighborhood who gave the shots twice weekly. Then I got brave and began giving them myself. A nutritional protocol was prescribed, and we also began improving Tim's diet. Tim was a good sport about taking a handful of pills a couple of times a day. Included in that mix of pills was nystatin, an antifungal medication. Skin testing showed a sensitivity to *Candida albicans*, and he had some classic symptoms of a systemic yeast problem: fatigue, foggy thinking, and food sensitivities (see Chapter 18). Our efforts to reduce sugars proved important, and we also found that certain artificial flavors and colors could quickly set off tics.

Cleaning up the home

I began making an effort to reduce dust in our home. We bought a dehumidifier to keep the mold count down. And we saw for ourselves that Tim did, indeed, have chemical sensitivities. When he used strong cleansers on his face or swam in a treated swimming pool, his eyes would start to roll. One day while with some friends, one of them was fooling around and accidentally sprayed a can of Raid, a pesticide, near Tim's face. He quickly retreated to his bedroom because his tics immediately intensified to the point of embarrassment.

Now I was convinced. I threw out scented candles and indoor and outdoor pesticides. We switched to nontoxic cleansers and bought unscented laundry and personal products.

The tics improved but remained quite strong for the first month, but soon the overall level was much less and a clear pattern emerged. We could almost always find the cause for what was triggering the tics. After about five months, when we stuck with the plan of dietary and nutritional changes, avoidance of allergens and toxic chemicals, and allergy therapy, the tics and other symptoms were virtually nonexistent.

Important lessons

A physician who doubted Tim's recovery suggested that he had just outgrown his tics. We know this was not the case. Three memorable events occurred well into his recovery that made it clear that the immune system and chemical sensitivities were involved. In the first incident, Tim was tic-free at the start of one day when he happened to step into a fire ant mound and received numerous bites. This immediately resulted in major tics that lasted approximately 24 hours. Another time he was again tic-free when he was inadvertently and directly exposed to overhead mosquito spraying while playing outside at night. This caused a frightening mood change and instant, severe tics. We quickly had him shower

> Another time he was again tic-free when he was inadvertently and directly exposed to overhead mosquito spraying while playing outside at night. This caused a frightening mood change and instant, severe tics.

and change clothes, and gave him an antihistamine. By late the next day, his symptoms had almost disappeared. Another chemical exposure took place when someone spilled paint thinner on his clothes at work. Tim had experienced no tics for months, but this caused a deep facial twitch to start that took two days to subside.

Without the opportunity to witness these three cause and effect reactions first hand, the sudden eruptions of symptoms would have seemed "mysterious," as if they happened randomly, just as the standard Tourette literature describes them. Each was a valuable lesson.

A major effort—but well worth it

This treatment plan was not easy. It took record-keeping, cajoling of the whole family to agree with the lifestyle changes, discipline, and determination. I brought Tim back for skin testing every six months because the tics started to increase slightly around that time, as if the treatment vials were not as effective anymore. After adjusting the concentrations of the substances in the vials, the symptoms were always further reduced. It was amazing! Not only did the tics go away with this treatment, but obsessive tendencies and mood swings disappeared as well.

It has been 14 years since Tim's recovery. He still watches his diet, takes nutrients, and avoids exposures to allergenic and toxic substances. We are incredibly grateful. He has an excellent job and is now socially secure. No one would ever suspect the nightmare we went through.

> *If you explore natural approaches for tics, we'd like to hear from you. Please contact us at: ACN, PO Box 2198, Broken Arrow, OK 74013 or by e-mail: srogers@latitudes.org. All reports are confidential.*

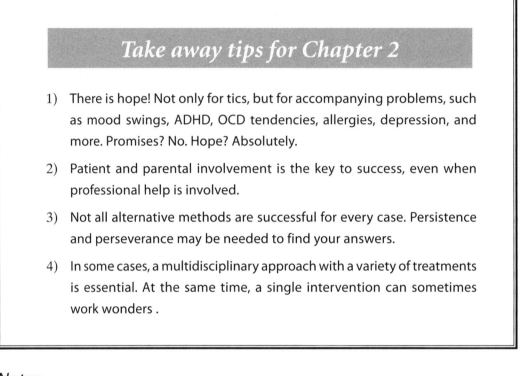

Take away tips for Chapter 2

1) There is hope! Not only for tics, but for accompanying problems, such as mood swings, ADHD, OCD tendencies, allergies, depression, and more. Promises? No. Hope? Absolutely.

2) Patient and parental involvement is the key to success, even when professional help is involved.

3) Not all alternative methods are successful for every case. Persistence and perseverance may be needed to find your answers.

4) In some cases, a multidisciplinary approach with a variety of treatments is essential. At the same time, a single intervention can sometimes work wonders .

Notes:

_____

_____

_____

_____

_____

_____

3

The Problem: Diagnosis
without Full Examination

ONE WEAKNESS IN THE TRADITIONAL MANNER of assessing tic conditions is that, typically, little effort is made to determine what is actually causing the symptoms. After ruling out other possible conditions, the prevailing approach is to match patient-reported symptoms to checklists for the purpose of providing a diagnosis. The next step is to consider medication needs, if any. Looking for biologic causes of the tics or possible aggravating factors is not standard medical practice. This approach reflects medical training and current conventional "best practices" on how to diagnose and manage tic disorders.

As new insights into the underlying causes of tics are uncovered, physicians will be more creative in helping patients control and prevent their tics. Many of these new clinical findings are discussed in this book.

Beyond "waxing and waning"

A person's tic symptoms usually change in severity or frequency, and/or they affect different muscles at different times. If you ask a specialist in movement disorders why this occurs, the usual response is, "This is what tics do—they come and they go. We call this waxing and waning." Most people dealing with tics soon learn to adopt this terminology to explain the symptoms. A mother might say to her husband about their son, "Billy's tics have been much worse this month. It must be the waxing and waning."

This term provides a false sense of understanding. It is a phrase that basically restates what the patient or caretaker already knows. Yes, tic symptoms tend to change in type, frequency, and severity over time. The key questions that should be asked are: Why are the tics worse or different at varying times, and what conditions allow symptoms to improve?

To answer these questions, it is important that physicians examine the patient's medical history, environmental history, nutritional status, and dietary habits, as well as any ongoing exposures to allergens or toxins. Ideally, this inquiry would also include maternal and patient issues that might be less obvious. This includes infections, vaccine history, dental work, the parents' health at the time of conception and the mother's health and environmental exposures. Intake of medications or supplements during pregnancy are also relevant. These are all important issues that are not usually investigated.

Healing the body to stop the tics

Coexisting physical complaints are often associated with tic disorders. Although there are conflicting reports on the incidence of allergy in tic disorders, Dr. C. S. Ho and fellow researchers report that allergy occurs at a significantly higher rate within the Tourette syndrome (TS) population than the general population. Furthermore, research shows that children with tic disorders—including both chronic motor tics and TS—have a higher number of other physical complaints than the normal population. These complaints include aches or pains, headaches, nausea, "feeling sick," stomachaches or cramps, and vomiting. Also, several studies document that those with TS have a tendency toward sleep-related problems, such as bedwetting, sleep talking, night terrors, difficulty falling asleep, and problems awakening. A fourfold increase in migraine headaches among those with TS was mentioned in Chapter 1. (Visual defects are also noted; see Chapter 10.)

One could argue that the experience of dealing with tics increases stress and anxiety and causes some children to experience one or more of the above problems. If this were the case, then the assumption would be that when the tics were controlled, the other physical complaints would lessen. However, researchers found that standard medication for tics did not reduce these types of symptoms.

Based on the investigations and clinical reports received by ACN, it would be wise to consider the full constellation of symptoms as clues to biologic dysfunction(s) that may also be at the root of the tics. People have reported to ACN that when they successfully used alternative or complementary treatments for tic disorders, not only did the tics subside, but accompanying physical symptoms were often reduced as well. Many times, problems that may coexist with tics, such as attention deficit disorder with hyperactivity (ADHD), obsessive-compulsive disorder (OCD), depression, anger control, and behavior problems, also tend to subside or disappear.

Investigate fully

Just as a person questions why they have a stomachache, a rash, or a backache, people should question and investigate why they have tics. Accepting or resigning oneself to the symptoms because "it runs in the family," or "my doctor said it's common, and I shouldn't worry about it," or "she will probably outgrow it," or "our psychiatrist told us it's genetic and the only option is drugs" does not invite useful inquiry that might open the door to true healing.

> Just as a person questions why they have a stomachache, a rash, or a backache, people should question and investigate why they have tics.

Frederic Speer, MD, author of the classic books *Handbook of Clinical Allergy: A Practical Guide to Patient Management* and *Food Allergy* pointed out that some conditions now considered allergic or immune-related diseases were once assumed to be of psychiatric origin. Dr. J. H. Rinkel, a leader in the development of allergy testing methods and treatment, emphasized the importance of fully questioning and exploring possible biologic causes when evaluating symptoms in a patient: "One must be taught to suspect, for if one does not suspect he does not test, and if he does not test he does not know."

Sidney M. Baker, MD, of Weston, Connecticut, is author of *Detoxification and Healing: The Key to Optimal Health* and coauthor of the development of a revolutionary, biomedical approach for reversing autism *(Autism: Effective Biomedical Treatments)*—a huge breakthrough for a condition that has baffled medical researchers. Dr. Baker summarized his basic approach for ACN: "By applying a simple kind of logic in which two questions are asked, I was able to forge ahead in the treatment of autism. Those two questions are: Is there something your body needs for which you have some individual, perhaps quirky, requirement that is not being met? Or, is there something you are getting that you as an individual have some quirky, sometimes unusual, need to avoid? It's pretty simple logic, but if you keep penetrating those questions, you can come up with things that are quite helpful to people."

> "Is there something your body needs for which you have some individual, perhaps quirky, requirement that is not being met? Or, is there something you are getting that you as an individual have some quirky, sometimes unusual, need to avoid?"
> —Sidney M. Baker, MD

The tic community could benefit from embracing the philosophies of Drs. Rinkel and Baker. The material in this book should encourage a more comprehensive way of looking at tics, and we hope that physicians will be more comfortable in searching for new causes and possible biologic and environmental triggers. The following chapters provide areas to explore as you seek to find the answers you need.

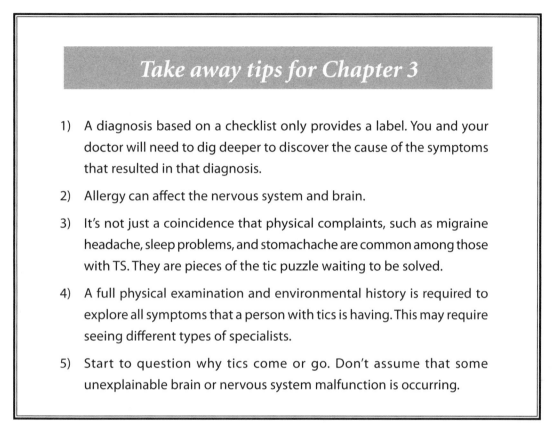

Take away tips for Chapter 3

1) A diagnosis based on a checklist only provides a label. You and your doctor will need to dig deeper to discover the cause of the symptoms that resulted in that diagnosis.

2) Allergy can affect the nervous system and brain.

3) It's not just a coincidence that physical complaints, such as migraine headache, sleep problems, and stomachache are common among those with TS. They are pieces of the tic puzzle waiting to be solved.

4) A full physical examination and environmental history is required to explore all symptoms that a person with tics is having. This may require seeing different types of specialists.

5) Start to question why tics come or go. Don't assume that some unexplainable brain or nervous system malfunction is occurring.

Notes:

_____

_____

_____

_____

_____

_____

SECTION TWO

Identifying Triggers for Tics

CHAPTER

4

ACN's Survey on Tic Triggers

YOU MAY HAVE HEARD THE QUESTION, "What makes her tick?" The spelling is different, but that's the issue! What *makes* a person tic? What accounts for the fact that symptoms are sometimes better and sometimes worse? This roller coaster pattern is actually encouraging because it means the body is capable of periods when tics are in relative remission.

The goal is to learn how to *extend* and *improve* those periods of remission and to *prevent* conditions that aggravate symptoms. Several years ago, ACN surveyed patients and families with tics and Tourette syndrome (TS) to gain information on any nonconventional therapies they were using. The results were published: "Nutritional Supplements and Complementary/Alternative Medicine in Tourette Syndrome" (*Journal of Child Adolescent Psychopharmacology* 2004;14:582–89). The information from this survey allowed us to develop logical areas to explore, and over the years we have discussed many of these natural treatments in our publication, *Latitudes* (now *Latitudes Online*; see page 274).

In 2003, ACN launched a different survey online to get feedback on personal triggers for tics—factors that can initiate or increase tic symptoms. The survey, which was concluded in 2004, documents that something as simple and common as orange juice, flashing lights, or the smell of perfume can make someone's tics worse.

The ACN survey

- ACN's Tic Triggers Survey was completed by 1,794 people worldwide and gives us new insight into the dynamics of tic symptoms. Participants were asked to select factors that they knew to set tics off or make them worse. Items were presented in two lists: dietary or ingested items (ranging from foods to medications), and classic environmental items (eg, dust or chlorine).

- A sophisticated program (Event Handler 2003; by UbiDog Productions) was used to allow only one completed survey per computer. The software recognized the Internet Protocol (the IP address—a unique 32-bit number). If someone completed the survey and then logged on to do it again, the second effort was blocked. This helped maintain the integrity of the data.

- Results of the survey are included in this chapter. This survey is not a scientific measure, but it does provide a valuable look at conditions that can contribute to tic symptoms for some people. The intent is to learn from each other and to raise awareness of the importance of dietary and environmental factors in tic symptoms.

- Participants were presented with online-lists of items and were asked to select those that had been found to be triggers for the case they were reporting on. The lists were developed from comments received from people who have contacted ACN and from previous surveys ACN has conducted. Participants could indicate "none" or "other," and they were invited to send additional observations by e-mail.

- Some of the categories were general in nature. For example, "sweets, sodas, and cane sugar" were grouped into the same category. The reason for this is that an observer can easily notice whether tics repeatedly increase after eating a candy bar or having a soft drink. Yet it can be more difficult to analyze whether a reaction is a direct result of exposure to corn syrup, honey, cane sugar, fructose, or another sweetener—any of which might have been used in the product. Additionally, other ingredients in a candy bar, such as chocolate or artificial coloring, could actually be the source of the problem, or a combination of items could be involved.

- Similarly, some people may realize that they react negatively to a strong chemical odor but have never differentiated their reaction to ammonia versus deodorizers, chlorine, or numerous cleansers. Again, a general response was requested. Only trials and careful observations over time can pinpoint specific causes for a person's symptoms.

- Seventy-one percent of those completing the survey did so on behalf of a relative, usually a child; 27% had tics themselves; 2% indicated a different relationship. The percentages of age groups in years reported on were: 0–5 (5%); 6–10 (34%); 11–15 (23%); 16–20 (7%); 21–35 (14%); 36–50 (11%); over 50 (6%).

Please note: Several widely recognized triggers for tics were not included in the survey because we were primarily seeking new ideas and trying to keep the list brief. These include fatigue and mental/emotional states, such as excitement, anxiety or worry, obsessiveness, fear, and self-consciousness. Some respondents considered these a type of stress.

Results of the ACN Survey on Tic Triggers
1,794 respondents (2003-2004)

The results of the survey are listed in order of frequency reported. The fact that items such as stress and caffeine, known triggers for tics, received a relatively high number of responses does not mean that they are potentially more detrimental than less frequently reported items, such as artificial colors, molds, or pesticides. It simply means that more people have made a connection between the items and symptoms.

1. Stress
2. Caffeine
3. Noise
4. Sweets/sodas/cane sugar
5. Alcohol
6. Video games
7. Infections (viral/bacterial)
8. Stimulant medications (ie, Ritalin)
9. Light (flashing, bright, or fluorescent)
10. Artificial colors
11. Car or bus rides
12. Clothing/fabric sensation on skin
13. Heat (temperature increase)
14. Specific foods (ie, corn, dairy, orange)
15. Artificial flavors
16. Cold medicines
17. Artificial sweeteners
18. Chemical exposures, (ie, cleaning products, formaldehyde, paint, gas fumes)
19. Dust
20. Molds
21. Preservatives (in foods)
22. Allergy medications
23. Personal scented products (ie, perfumes, cologne, aftershave)
24. Smoke/smoking
25. Air fresheners (plug-in type, spray, and other forms)
26. Pollens
27. Dental work
28. Monosodium glutamate (MSG)
29. Candles (scented)/potpourri
30. Carpeting (new)
31. Pesticides
32. Cell phone use
33. Hepatitis B vaccine

Note: *Number of respondents indicating that a specific item above was problematic ranged from 1,164 (stress) to 35 (hepatitis B vaccine). Responses for alcohol were prorated to include patients 21 years or older. Fourteen percent reported no environmental triggers and 35% indicated no known dietary triggers.*

Other Reported Tic Triggers

Some additional triggers reported to ACN are listed here, in alphabetical order. It is possible to have other triggers that are not listed either here or on the opposite page.

- Carpeting, removal
- Computer use
- Doing nothing (bored)
- Emotional issues
- Feeling hungry
- Fragrance of flowers
- Hand-holding
- Having a head cold
- Insect bites
- Listening to someone talk about tics
- Obsessive thoughts that cause anxiety
- Other food additives

- Seasonal changes
- Seeing other people's tics
- Shampoo for dandruff/ eczema
- Smoke odors (lingering)
- Stadiums or amusement parks at night (lights)
- Temperature changes (rapid) in either direction
- Watching television or a movie, especially in a dark room or theater (see reminder below)

Important Reminder

These trigger reports are preliminary. If only a small number of people communicated on a certain item, this does not mean it is not a potential trigger for a large number of people. It may simply reflect that the particular item was not carefully considered. Watching television and movies is a good example. We did not include these in the survey because we accepted the popular theory within the tic community that children have more symptoms while watching TV because they are relaxing and "letting the tics out." Since the survey, we have learned that the light frequency from screens can trigger tics. Once this finding is more widely recognized, observations of people with tics during times of computer use or while watching television/movies can be expected to increase. Please see Chapter 10 for a discussion of screens and photosensitivity.

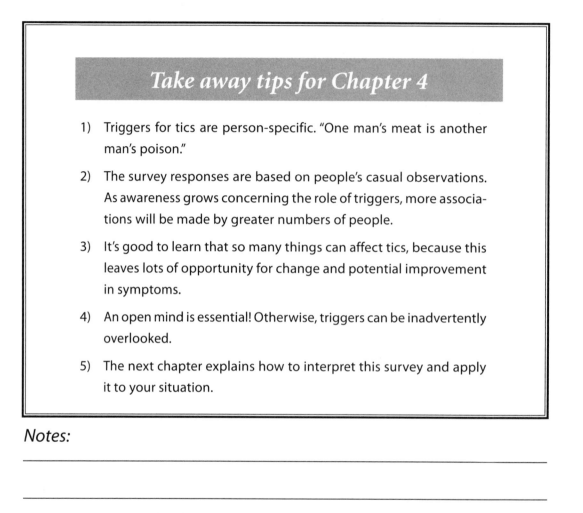

Take away tips for Chapter 4

1) Triggers for tics are person-specific. "One man's meat is another man's poison."

2) The survey responses are based on people's casual observations. As awareness grows concerning the role of triggers, more associations will be made by greater numbers of people.

3) It's good to learn that so many things can affect tics, because this leaves lots of opportunity for change and potential improvement in symptoms.

4) An open mind is essential! Otherwise, triggers can be inadvertently overlooked.

5) The next chapter explains how to interpret this survey and apply it to your situation.

Notes:

_____

_____

_____

_____

_____

_____

_____

CHAPTER

5

Understanding Survey Results

NOW THAT WE HAVE THE ACN TIC TRIGGERS SURVEY RESULTS (described in Chapter 4), interpreting them is the next step. The first thing to understand is that the survey—the first of its kind—is a starting point toward better insight into the role of triggers in tic disorders. The results were collected informally and cannot be considered an absolute "snapshot" that defines the entire tic community. Yet, the survey responses provide new and valuable information that will transform the way tic disorders are managed. (We are grateful to all who took time to participate!)

It is safe to assume that survey respondents often underestimated the number of triggers involved. In other words, some trigger responses went unobserved and unreported by those completing the survey. The following are some of the reasons for this tendency:

- *It's a new concept:* Many people have never considered looking for triggers for their tics. As this approach is not standard medical protocol, doctors do not recommend this be done. Some patients and families have probably not thought about issues beyond stress, excitement, fatigue, and caffeine. At the time when the survey was completed, most responses were likely based on past awareness, with the majority of triggers never having been investigated.

- *Parents were responding for children:* Many respondents were parents completing the survey on behalf of children. Sometimes a parent can observe a cause and effect reaction (exposure to a tic trigger and onset of tics) easily, but on other occasions, if the parent did not specifically question the child, it would not be clear that a particular situation or item was to blame for an onset or increase in tics. Furthermore, the child may not have made the connection or even paid attention to the tics (see next point).

- *Adults—much less children—are not always aware of their own tics!* Interesting research by Pappert and associates revealed that half of adult participants who considered themselves to be tic-free were actually experiencing tics, as documented on videotape. Clearly, someone not tuned into his or her own tics is also much less able to notice tic triggers.

- *Environmental factors can overlap:* Exposure to multiple tic triggers at the same time makes specific reactions difficult to isolate or identify without professional help.

- *Hypersensitivities can be difficult to ascertain:* Once someone becomes hypersensitive to toxic chemicals, standard allergens, or foods, very low levels of that substance can cause a reaction. The amount of a substance can be so minimal that its presence may not be detected, yet the body reacts.

- *Stress affects level of response:* When the immune system is relatively strong and the central nervous system less stressed, a person might not react to a given stimulus. But when that person is tired, overstressed, or "overexposed" to toxic substances, a reaction occurs more readily. This can be difficult to sort out.

- *"Masking" adds to the challenge:* A phenomenon known as *masking* makes it difficult to tell when a substance is a problem for the body. Masking means that the body is so accustomed to the substance that it has adapted to it in the sense that symptoms are not clearly associated with it. This phenomenon can be better understood in the context of an elimination diet (where substances thought to cause allergic reactions are removed from the diet). When a problem food is being consumed regularly, recognizing its role in causing chronic symptoms, such as fatigue or foggy thinking, is difficult. When that food is completely avoided for an extended period, then purposefully eaten, a clear reaction will usually be seen, if a sensitivity exists. Another example would be sensitivity to a perfume; people with this sensitivity could be accustomed to such an exposure on a daily basis and never connect that exposure with the symptoms it is causing. If they were to live in a scent-free environment for an extended period and then be re-exposed to a strong dose of perfume, they might be able to make the connection. Masking affects the survey because it results in having many aggravating stimuli go unrecognized.

- *Additives may be hidden:* It is often difficult to know the source of ingredients in foods, such as "natural flavorings" which, by federal law, can be derived from any number of foods.

- *Observation of many items is not possible or consistent across age groups:* Some items do not lend themselves to common observation. For example, "new carpeting" was on the survey list, but not everyone responding to the survey would have an opportunity to observe a reaction to odors and toxins from new carpeting. Similarly, stimulant medication would have been taken by only a portion of respondents, and pesticides—a potential trigger—are often applied in public settings without occupants being informed. Young children are less likely than adults to report an increase in tics from cell phones because they use them less, and adults are exposed to video games less frequently than children. All these types of issues affect how an individual would respond to the survey.

For the reasons just discussed, more people are assumed to be affected by a wider range of triggers than survey results indicate. As an acknowledgment of this disparity, the results on page 62 are presented in order of the frequency of survey responses received, and percentages of responses were not included, as they would be misleading.

An example of results underrepresenting the occurrence of triggers

Heat is one environmental, or sensory factor that has been formally studied as related to tics. Research showed that 24% of adults participating in a survey reported increased tics on exposure to heat. In a laboratory setting with adult males, there was a general increase in tics associated with the sweat rate when the temperature was raised, and this tic increase was prominent among 50% of the group. Yet, results of the ACN Tic Triggers Survey indicate that only 12% of respondents chose "increased heat" as a trigger. This percentage is clearly much lower than the published research findings. We believe such underrepresenting is typical of respondents' lack of awareness of triggers as reflected in the ACN survey.

Playing detective—a baseball game example

Several reactions to triggers can occur at the same time, making it difficult for parents and children to understand which one is responsible for an increase in tics. For example, a child's tics might significantly increase while playing in a baseball game because the youngster is:

- Playing directly in the bright sun (light sensitivity);
- Experiencing an increase in outdoor temperature or an increase in body temperature from exercise;
- Reacting to sugary or artificially-enhanced drinks provided by the coach;
- Feeling irritated by the texture of the uniform;
- Being stressed by the pressures or excitement of the game; or
- Having an allergic reaction to kicked-up dirt, freshly cut grass, or grass contaminated with chemical fertilizers or pesticides.

The fact is, any or all of these factors could potentially be involved in heightening a tic response. (This is not to imply that there is always a readily understandable cause.)

Why bother searching?

The main purpose of identifying environmental insults that aggravate tics is so that they can be avoided whenever possible, and appropriate interventions can be started to address the sensitivity.

Trigger information is also important when conducting studies. Researchers who have been unaware of the connection between the immediate environment, diet, and tics may have unwittingly had study results thrown off. For example, a "controlled" study for a tic medication, in which the researcher assumes the only significant change taking place is the use of the drug, takes on a different meaning when significant environmental or dietary factors that can impact tics are considered. This issue is particularly relevant in studies with a small number of subjects.

> The main purpose of identifying environmental insults that aggravate tics is so that they can be avoided whenever possible, and appropriate interventions can be started to address the sensitivity.

The challenge of identifying triggers

Consider what happens when someone has an outbreak of hives. Hives are known to be an immune response to some environmental/dietary factors, yet allergists will tell you that in most cases the actual cause of the hives goes undetected, even with careful investigation.

Finding triggers for chronic tics can be more complex than tracking down the source of a sporadic case of hives. It takes effort, and all efforts may not be successful. Yet, when the culprits are identified, the rewards are immeasurable.

In the next chapter you will learn more by reading letters received by our organization that describe some of the triggers others have discovered, and you will see how these discoveries can lead to a reduction of tic symptoms.

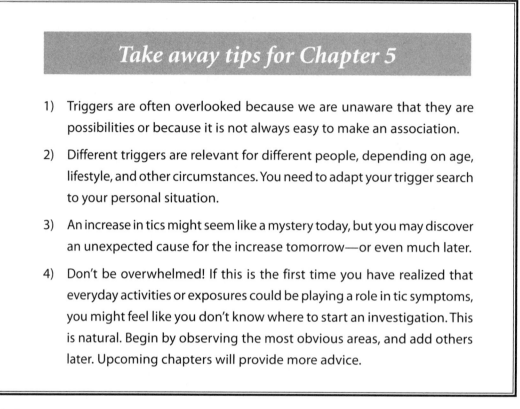

Take away tips for Chapter 5

1) Triggers are often overlooked because we are unaware that they are possibilities or because it is not always easy to make an association.

2) Different triggers are relevant for different people, depending on age, lifestyle, and other circumstances. You need to adapt your trigger search to your personal situation.

3) An increase in tics might seem like a mystery today, but you may discover an unexpected cause for the increase tomorrow—or even much later.

4) Don't be overwhelmed! If this is the first time you have realized that everyday activities or exposures could be playing a role in tic symptoms, you might feel like you don't know where to start an investigation. This is natural. Begin by observing the most obvious areas, and add others later. Upcoming chapters will provide more advice.

Notes:

_____

_____

_____

_____

_____

_____

CHAPTER

6

Letters on Triggers

THE FOLLOWING LETTERS received by ACN highlight numerous factors that can affect tic symptoms. We hope this sampling from patients and those close to them will help readers identify factors aggravating their disorder and ways to address them. As this book emphasizes, that which increases or improves symptoms for one person may not affect someone else. Among those who initiated interventions, some had quick and dramatic results, while others reported more moderate and gradual improvement, even when undertaking similar efforts. Letters have been edited for clarity and space.

❖

I have Tourette syndrome and have found that nondrug, dietary management is far more effective than drugs in controlling my tics. Besides being ineffective, the medication I tried had horrible side effects. Therefore, I now control my symptoms simply by being very careful about what I eat. For example, I do not eat anything that contains refined sugar. This is very difficult and requires that I check ingredients in bread, sauces, savory dishes, drinks (including alcoholic drinks), and medications taken for other problems—everything. It is, however, definitely worth the effort because I am so much better and have eliminated almost all tics.

I used to have very severe motor tics, vocalizations, coprolalia (uncontrollable swearing), echolalia (repeating phrases or words), touching, mimicking, self-injurious behaviors, and compulsions. The worst symptoms I had to endure were the motor tics and coprolalia. Now I feel almost normal! If I accidentally eat sugar, I get the tics back for a few days. I have to be especially careful with fruit juices; some manufacturers in England put sugar into their "pure" fruit juices. (I can eat fruit and milk—things that naturally contain sugar.) I discovered this reaction myself by trial and error.

Many people comment on how much better I am. It annoys me, however, that they often don't believe me when I tell them the reason (dietary changes) for my improvement. They suggest that I simply "outgrew" my TS, or make comments that imply that I have imagined having TS or that I've had a "faith cure." I am a 26-year-old woman with a scientific background and careful mind, and I know, based on observation and deduction, that the lifestyle changes I made affected my disorder. I'm so happy that the Association for Comprehensive NeuroTherapy is recognizing the benefits of a dietary/allergy approach to relieving the symptoms of tic disorders. I'm a great believer in curing problems at their root rather than clumsily attempting to target symptoms with drugs.

> I am a 26-year-old woman with a scientific background and careful mind, and I know, based on observation and deduction, that the lifestyle changes I made affected my disorder.

�֎

Triggers for my ten-year-old son's tics include dust, mold, and fall pollens. A few foods are also a problem; corn, dairy products, MSG, and pumpkin seeds. We find that when we keep these things under control, he is tic-free.

✖

During time in a naturopathic clinic in Oregon, we saw a 12-year-old boy whose parents had stopped his medical treatment for Tourette's in favor of an alternative approach. His prior treatment had consisted of clonidine, which suppressed his outbursts, but had, in the words of his father, "turned him into a zombie." The clinicians ordered laboratory work and recommended that the boy be taken off sugary foods and similar products. He was found to have high levels of both copper and cadmium. Select vitamin, mineral, and chelating amino acid supplements (to help remove toxic metals from the body) were prescribed. One year later, the patient was still in treatment, but he now had only a slight facial tic instead of the "72 outbursts in 50 minutes" that his teacher had recorded.

✢

I am a 36-year-old male who has had symptoms of Tourette's since the age of eight. My triggers include flashing lights and flickering fluorescent bulbs. A sudden change in temperature (such as coming in from the cold and immediately washing my hands in hot water) will also cause a tic. Any flashing light is sufficient to trigger my tics, but police car emergency lights, in particular, affect me because of the red and blue hypnotic and blinding pulse light. Yellow and slower rotating lights don't assault my nerves as badly.

I used to have migraine headaches and was so light sensitive that I could detect fluctuations in fluorescent bulbs—almost a visible shudder of the light-wave hitting me; fortunately, newer bulbs are not as bad. I was once pulled over in North Carolina by a police car with a fast "popping" sort of red and white light, and a blinding fierce blue light. (I had done nothing wrong—they simply wanted to inform me of something.) I started thrashing so violently in my seat that when the officer came to shine his flashlight in my face, he called for an ambulance. Once I was able to communicate that the problem was the lights, they switched them off, and the tics subsided.

✢

We have found tics can be reduced dramatically by eliminating food additives from the diet. The worst ones in our case are artificial flavors (including vanillin), artificial colors, such as Red Dye #40, Yellow #5, and the preservatives BHT, BHA, and TBHQ.

✤

I'm a 42-year-old man who served as a medical technician in the service and in civilian life for ten years. I suffered from the embarrassment of TS all my life.

About 15 years ago, I changed my eating habits because of other health problems. I drastically reduced refined foods and red meat and began eating more raw fruits and vegetables. I also began taking nutritional supplements. This diet changed my life, and my TS symptoms were vastly improved. However, it wasn't until I stopped consuming corn syrup and, especially, high-fructose corn syrup, that my symptoms almost entirely subsided. Corn syrup is in many food items, and, therefore, I must read the labels carefully.

Don't think this is "all in my head." I am well aware of the placebo effect and can assure you that this was not the case. Please don't let this letter end up in a wastebasket. I feel strongly that others could be helped.

✤

When I was a child, my tics and other health anomalies were never addressed. As the years went on, it became increasingly difficult to live with my tic disorder. It was especially embarrassing to have dinner at a restaurant. Just getting the spoon to my mouth was a horrendous chore.

In my 20s, I noticed that stress, caffeine, and candy exacerbated a neck jerk. In my 50s, I finally eliminated smoking and coffee, and the head-shaking subsided. I then began eating a macrobiotic diet and since then have eaten only organic foods and no sugar, alcohol, or caffeine. I eat homemade vegetarian foods that don't contain chemicals or yeast. Chemicals and stimulants are poison to people with tics.

I still have to work with my tics and tremors, but having eliminated these substances, there is a far better chance of controlling them. Please look into this way of eating. Over time, you will see that chemically-saturated foods or other particular foods can affect the nervous system unfavorably. I know! This has been my lifelong struggle. Perhaps my experience can aid others.

✢

Our adult son is addicted to smoking, and we see how this adversely affects his tics. In addition, I watched one day as he cleaned his bedroom. He was removing books from the bookcase; this hadn't been done in a very long time and I could see dust flying around in the air. His tics really flared up from the exposure to dust. I never knew dust could make tics worse.

✢

My daughter (six years old) has attention deficit disorder with hyperactivity and severe food intolerances. She developed tics immediately after being given Ritalin. They were severe and included eye-rolling, head jerking sideways, face-stretching, and vocalizations. She has been off Ritalin for four months now but still has bouts of tics. We have found that removing certain foods from her diet greatly improves control of her symptoms, and when we reintroduce these foods, the symptoms, including obsessive-compulsive behaviors, tics, eczema, rashes, moodiness, and bowel/bladder disturbances, return. About three days after the problem food is removed from her diet, the symptoms subside once again.

✢

I am severely allergic to ragweed. Other problem allergens are grasses, house dust, dust mites, and mold. I have suffered terribly with tics all my life. After seeing an environmental physician and getting treated for these allergies, I hardly have any tics for the first time ever. I also learned from this doctor that I have food allergies, and I now watch my diet and take several nutrients that he prescribed. Someone who knows me recently asked if I even have tics anymore! If I go off the allergy and supplement program, however, tics start to come back.

�֎

I have found that when my son eats peanut butter, his complex vocal and motor tics increase greatly.

✖

Tourette syndrome was diagnosed in my son at three years of age. He is now six years old. At one point, we stopped medications and tried altering his diet. We've learned that sugars, sodas, chocolate, and starchy foods bring on his main tic: circling and throwing his arms and hands about. During the winter holidays, we weren't selective in what he ate and, therefore, the tics and accompanying frustration greatly increased. (I can't tell you how often I've been told incorrectly that food and exposure to given stimuli does not make a difference!)

✖

We went to an environmental physician and started my son on an elimination diet. The tics practically disappeared—they were at least 90% improved. I couldn't believe it! Then we started adding foods back into the diet and discovered that sugar was the number-one offender.

✖

My son was on Haldol for Tourette syndrome symptoms but, after some time, it was no longer helpful. He is now on Orap, which controls most of his tics. One day after shopping he bought a cola at a local store. As soon as he finished it, his head started bobbing, and he gulped repeatedly. After trial and error, I realized that colas made him tic more.

✖

Eliminating allergens has helped with our son's tics. We removed our carpets, got rid of a down comforter, and have done battle with bathroom mold. Eliminating artificial colors and flavors, dairy, and corn syrup as best as we could helped with behavior. His lip-licking tics (the most obvious) which for the past six years have tended to be worse in the fall until the first frost, were not as pronounced this past fall. Tenex (guanfacine hydrochloride; a blood pressure medication prescribed to control tics) seemed to make my son weepy and aggressive. A couple of years ago, after reading Daniel G. Amen's book *Healing ADHD*, I agreed to a trial of Prozac. The results of Prozac on behavior have been pretty dramatic. We could throw away the sticker charts used for behavior modification as our son was more compliant and less moody. Things have gotten increasingly better socially. This summer for the first time, the neighborhood kids are ringing our doorbell. Last week he said he was having the "best week of my life, because the kids like me." I am convinced there's some sort of allergy link to his tics. We have found our answer by combining traditional drug therapy with nonconventional approaches.

⁕

Many of us with Tourette's have a "punny" sense of humor. My mind is always looking for any chance for some word-play. I read in publications by your organization that perfumes and scented products can be triggers for tics. I already knew that a strong perfume scent could aggravate my tics. I'm a clerk at a Canadian post office, and one night I was sorting bundles of magazines entitled *Cosmetics*. I was looking at this title word on cover after cover. Then my Tourettic mind started looking at it from a different angle. I saw the title become "cos-me-tics," pronounced "cause me tics." And it's true—they can cos me tics!

⁕

When my son was nine years old, a neuroleptic medication was prescribed for his severe tics. (Neuroleptics are tranquilizers and antipsychotic drugs). This calmed him down so that he stopped hurting himself. His head-jerking, shoulder and body jerks, eye-blinking and rolling eyes, snorting, yelping, whooping, cursing, and repeating things all slowed down. However, the drug made him listless, and under stress, the same symptoms would reappear. The neurologist attempted to reduce his dosage, but the symptoms returned every time. I began to study nutrition and took him off sodas, Kool-Aid, candy, chocolate, ice cream (which would make him totally wild), boxed cereal with sugar, processed foods with preservatives, and any kind of junk food. I supplemented with a good multivitamin and gave him extra magnesium and calcium. All of this seemed to work, so I slowly decreased his medicine until he completely stopped taking it. He has improved by leaps and bounds, and the tic symptoms have slowly disappeared.

✢

Our daughter had tics for seven years (she's now 13 years old). These have included facial and vocal tics. She would bite herself until she was black and blue. She also had night terrors, panic attacks, and irrational fears. After she underwent allergy testing, we took her off all wheat, corn, milk, and soy. She was tic-free. Then we reintroduced these foods into her diet one by one to test her reaction. She had the worst reaction when she was challenged with wheat. Several facial tics appeared immediately, and she became irritable and sleepy.

✢

The tic disorder PANDAS has been diagnosed in my seven-year-old son. We have noticed that television is clearly a trigger, especially the "japanimation" variety of cartoon type shows, such as, "YuGiOH" and "Pokemon." Other types of shows are not as bad for him as these. Once we noticed this triggering, we limited TV viewing to 30 minutes.

Television viewing would make his tics start up immediately. Both complex motor tics and vocal tics would get going—sometimes as frequent as one per second. It was so heartbreaking to observe that I often had to leave the room while the TV was on. He could be looking at the TV, ticcing like crazy, then turn away from it and hold a conversation for a few minutes with almost no tics, then turn back to the TV, and ticcing would start again.

After reading suggestions included in your interactive forum on *www.Latitudes.org,* we eliminated watching television completely for several weeks. We also eliminated milk from the diet and began taking supplements. Tics improved greatly. When we went back to allowing TV, we used a flat-screen LCD monitor (liquid crystal display; see Chapter 10), and we limited our son's viewing time to 15 minutes. Although he would still have minor eye squints, there were no complex motor tics or any vocal tics. It was quite a change. We have had one exposure to a standard CRT (cathode ray tube) TV screen during the last several weeks. During that half hour, I saw several tics begin that included throat-clearing, cough, leg jerk, and some eye rolls. These had not occurred for one month or so, and they were clearly a reaction to that exposure.

> We have had one exposure to a standard CRT (cathode ray tube) TV screen during the last several weeks. During that half hour, I saw several tics begin that included throat-clearing, cough, leg jerk, and some eye rolls. These had not occurred for one month or so, and they were clearly a reaction to that exposure.

I was the last person who would believe that alternative approaches could have helped his disorder. In the past, I'd always been quick to ask for antibiotics or other standard medical treatment. I was in a desperate state when PANDAS was diagnosed, but your website gave us such hope. Over time, we learned that our son needed to have his immune system strengthened, so we stopped feeding him foods that were disrupting his health, and we began to manage his triggers by making needed changes in his environment. The result has been unbelievable, and I am truly thankful.

✣

My son came home from school on Monday ticcing intensely and displaying obsessive-compulsive symptoms that we had never seen before. When I checked on what he had eaten at school, nothing seemed amiss—but then he told me of the strong smell that came from new carpeting in his classroom. I checked, and sure enough, new carpeting was laid in my son's classroom over a long weekend. The school finally moved the class until the room had been thoroughly aired. Interestingly, the teacher had noticed that the kids with ADHD were also much more hyper from the new carpeting exposure.

We have seen similar temporary reactions in our son to all strong-smelling household cleaners, gasoline, pesticides, and other items. As a result, we have gone as "natural" as possible in our home.

✢

My eight-year-old daughter's tics were so bad that they were driving her crazy. I was devastated. She developed many types of tics, and they were constant. A doctor gave us a prescription medication for the tics, but we never filled it. After communicating with ACN several months ago, we cleaned dust from the home, bought her an allergy-free pillow, and began using unscented laundry detergent. We also stopped using fabric softener and stopped burning candles. I started my daughter on a nutrient program. The results have been miraculous. Her tics are now few and far between. I want to thank you for your help and for your publication (*Latitudes*). You have had a great impact on our lives. (See page 274 for information on *Latitudes,* now *Latitudes Online.*)

✢

I have been experimenting with food additives related to the occurrence of my son's tics. The preservatives, BHA and BHT, and the artificial sweetener, NutraSweet (aspartame), are the worst offenders.

✢

Our son was treated with Haldol and Orap for TS, but the drugs did not control symptoms; he had severe tics and vocalizations even with the drugs. In addition, he became depressed and had mood swings along with attention difficulties. He was gaining weight steadily as a side effect of the medication and had reached a point where he would not even go out in public. I repeatedly asked the doctor if foods or sugars could have anything to do with Tourette's and was repeatedly told they did not.

One day I saw the "Donahue" program that featured Doris J. Rapp, MD, an environmental physician. The show included a guest in whom TS had been diagnosed. He was about my son's age. This guest had allergies to certain foods, including sugar and certain chemicals. An allergy treatment and change in the guest's diet controlled his symptoms! After seeing the show, we went to an environmental allergist, and my son has since made tremendous progress. We watch my son faithfully now for any reaction to food. We've found that NutraSweet causes tics, hyperactivity, excessive body heat, and irritability. Monosodium glutamate (MSG) and sodium nitrate cause personality and mood changes. We have implemented the allergist's recommendations for more than two years, and my son is doing very well. He works hard to control his health, and no one meeting him would know he has a tic disorder.

I am a 53-year-old woman and have had symptoms of obsessive-compulsive behavior and a tendency toward movement disorders since early childhood. Triggers include cigarette smoke, certain chemicals, and select foods. Fluorescent lighting and proximity to electrical equipment and generators trigger symptoms as well.

Traditional doctors in my area ignore the fact that my child's symptoms worsen around (treated) swimming pools or following insect bites. Some other triggers for my son's tics are scented candles, dust, mold, orange juice, strawberries, artificial flavors and colors, MSG, and artificial sweeteners.

I am an adult with ADHD and TS, and am president of a local support Tourette syndrome chapter. I have learned that life is a balancing act. High-fructose corn syrup, refined sugars such as that on coated cereals, soda pop, etc, can send someone like me into oblivion.

While remodeling our home, we pulled up an old carpet (moldy and dusty). Our nine-year-old son suddenly developed such severe tics that we had to take him to the hospital emergency room. We have since learned a great deal about his allergies. In our case, there has been a definite benefit from environmental medicine.

✢

Television viewing and computer exposure are sure triggers for my son. We experimented and found that he was helped greatly by eliminating screen viewing. His problem behaviors and tics were reduced significantly by this intervention. At first I was intimidated at the idea of eliminating television viewing and computer use, but our children did not mind, and our house became so much quieter. The kids played together more, and we began doing more things together as a family including spending time at the park, playing board games, and reading.

Since that time, we have changed many other things to help him, the most significant being beginning him on a food elimination diet to determine sensitivities and giving him vitamins and essential fatty acids. After removing milk, corn, eggs, and chocolate from my son's diet and starting him on a supplement program guided by a naturopathic doctor and our pediatrician, he was again able to tolerate the screen viewing.

✢

How I wish I had learned about alternative treatments before our son, Pete, was medicated for severe tics. He had terrible reactions to the first drug. The second one merely made him tired and did not relieve the tics. We saw 12 doctors and not one of them informed us of the side effects of these drugs. Had we known, we would not have given the drugs to our son. In addition, not one physician mentioned possible "triggers" that we could have explored.

At one point a doctor prescribed Ritalin, although an evaluation noted that my son did not have an attention deficit disorder. I agreed to allow my son to receive the drug because, at the time, I did not want to appear to be uncooperative. The Ritalin made

Pete nuts! Soon after I gave him his first dose he ran around like a maniac. Thank goodness the drug had a brief effect in his body. He "crashed" that night, and I never gave it to him again.

I began reading information posted online and started down an alternative path. I have never looked back. While I am heartened to hear that standard medication can be an answer for some people, it was an awful experience for us.

My son has always been a spring allergies/asthma kid. I find that his food sensitivities are worse in the spring, and he also tics more in the spring. This spring his tics are the best they have been in four years. I think the efforts we have made to build his immune system with supplements, dietary changes, and environmental adjustments have helped in healing his body. It is my opinion that medication should only be used once all other efforts have been made, such as ruling out PANDAS, adjusting the diet, exploring vitamin deficiencies, and initiating a trial of avoiding visual flicker through TV and computer screens. We have also found craniosacral therapy and reflexology helpful, and Pete loves these treatments.

> He had terrible reactions to the first drug. The second one merely made him tired and did not relieve the tics. We saw 12 doctors and not one of them informed us of the side effects of these drugs. Had we known, we would not have given the drugs to our son. In addition, not one physician mentioned possible "triggers" that we could have explored.

�֞

I have major tics. Heat, humidity, and direct sun can turn me into a basket case.

✖

We have just finished our food elimination diet. When we were reintroducing certain foods, we learned that my son reacted to dairy with increased motor tics, vocal tics, hyperactivity, and impulsiveness. By far, dairy products were the worst for him. When fed eggs, he was more emotional and had motor tics. Chocolate made him very hyper. Corn also aggravated tics, and he was impulsive and emotional. (He seemed fine after having soy and wheat.) The corn allergy really surprised me; I don't think I would have picked up on this if we had not done the food elimination diet. It seems corn is in everything!

✦

I am 30 years old and have had a serious case of obsessive-compulsive disorder (OCD) since I was six. About one year ago, I stopped eating dairy products to see whether I could clear up a rash. Three days after making this change, I noticed that the number of obsessive thoughts and compulsions I was having declined by approximately 70%. This improvement lasted as long as I did not consume any dairy products. Then about one month later, I had ice cream, a cheese sandwich, and yogurt, all in the same afternoon. That night, all the symptoms of OCD returned with full force. I then began to experiment with other foods.

I discovered that I am allergic to most common allergens and that when I eliminate all of these things from my diet, I am entirely symptom-free. I now realize that many other mental and physical symptoms I have had throughout my life were also caused by allergies. Some of these symptoms include irritability, short-term memory loss, insomnia, muscle aches, eczema, and even mild, dream-like hallucinations. I begin to experience symptoms one or two hours after having eaten something to which I am allergic and continue to have symptoms for up to 48 hours. All this has made me wonder whether some of the people living in mental institutions only have conditions caused by something as simple as allergens.

> This improvement lasted as long as I did not consume any dairy products. Then about one month later, I had ice cream, a cheese sandwich, and yogurt, all in the same afternoon. That night, all the symptoms of OCD returned with full force. I then began to experiment with other foods.

Because I am allergic to so many common foods, such as wheat, corn, nuts, beans, tomatoes, potatoes, and some other items, it is difficult to avoid these foods all of the time. Fortunately, however, I have been able to learn a lot about how I react to particular foods. This knowledge has given me a great deal more control over my life and a sense of new confidence. I have learned, for example, that products containing vanilla cause symptoms of hypochondria. Corn products, on the other hand, make me irritable and often cause me to have trouble sleeping.

I have since learned that the idea of an association between OCD and allergies has been around for many years, but no studies have been done. I would advise people wishing to explore a possible link between a mental disorder and allergies to first investigate foods and chemicals to which they may be allergic. Then they must carefully read the ingredients of every food they ingest. The book, *No More Allergies* by Gary Null contains a section on brain allergies and has been a wonderful resource for me.

❖

My name is Martine Fornoville, and I am president of the Hamilton Chapter of the Tourette Syndrome Foundation in Ontario, Canada.

As I filled out the ACN Tic Triggers Survey (see Chapter 4), I checked off an almost ridiculous number of answers, purely because I have such difficulties with sensory over-stimulation issues in all senses:

Visually: Lights present a major problem for me—when they are too bright or there are flashing lights, strobe lights, or anything bright that changes color quickly;

Aurally: Loud sounds—such as movie theatre "surround sounds," loud and throbbing music—overstimulate me very easily;

Sense of touch: Clothing and anything that touches me, including human contact, frequently starts me writhing; textures felt by my hands or through my mouth bother me. I simply cannot tolerate certain foods purely because of the thought of their texture. (It's enough to make me gag!);

Temperature sensitivities: For myself and many of the kids with whom I work, heat sensitivity is a huge issue. For example, in the dead of winter, an 18-year-old who had Tourette's showed up wearing sandals and no socks;

Sense of smell: Cleaning products, smoke, perfumes, paint, gas fumes, exhaust, and specific foods have an intense effect on me; and

Finally, the "mind" sense: Having too much on my mind, the overstimulation of attention, and difficulties with impulse control, can be environmental triggers.

✧

My son is very aware of physical touch and can become aggravated or distressed by it. He says when he feels this way, it makes him tic more. We have cut tags out of all his clothes for years because he can't stand that sensation. We now buy him soft cotton clothing and sheets. He is even bothered by touching the fuzz on a peach skin.

✧

Completing a food elimination diet was the number one best thing we could have done for my son. I am now able to rotate corn, eggs and chocolate back into his diet, but milk still sends him into a tailspin. The only time he tics now is when he drinks milk, which also has the effect of making his behavior intolerable. I am a huge believer in starting with a food elimination diet. Our pediatrician questioned whether the effort of doing this was worth the try. Well, let me tell you that no matter how hard eliminating some foods from our diet has been, it is not nearly as hard as dealing with the tics and behavioral issues.

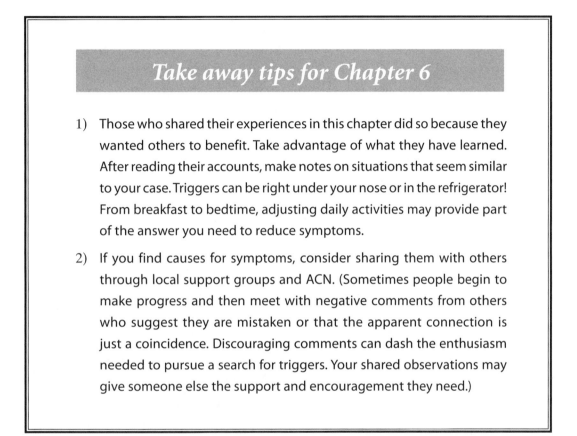

Take away tips for Chapter 6

1) Those who shared their experiences in this chapter did so because they wanted others to benefit. Take advantage of what they have learned. After reading their accounts, make notes on situations that seem similar to your case. Triggers can be right under your nose or in the refrigerator! From breakfast to bedtime, adjusting daily activities may provide part of the answer you need to reduce symptoms.

2) If you find causes for symptoms, consider sharing them with others through local support groups and ACN. (Sometimes people begin to make progress and then meet with negative comments from others who suggest they are mistaken or that the apparent connection is just a coincidence. Discouraging comments can dash the enthusiasm needed to pursue a search for triggers. Your shared observations may give someone else the support and encouragement they need.)

Notes:

_____

_____

_____

_____

_____

7

Your Search for Triggers

AN OPEN MIND IS CRITICAL WHEN EXPLORING possible factors that may be making tics worse. The ACN Tic Triggers Checklist in this chapter provides many of the possibilities. You may find it helpful to review the list at intervals. A factor that doesn't seem like a possible issue now may reveal itself later.

See Sections Four and Five of this book for an understanding of how items on the list could be affecting symptoms. The more educated you are about tic triggers before you begin your investigation, the better your chances for success. If you suspect a potential trigger, write it down and begin careful observations.

Sometimes you will find a trigger by removing that item and watching to see what happens in its absence; for example, you take all foods that contain artificial additives out of the diet and by doing so you see an improvement in tics. Other times, you will learn by observing a negative response after an exposure, such as when a person is sensitive to food additives but eats something containing them and symptoms flare. You may need professional help to find all the answers you need.

Using the ACN Tic Triggers Checklist

The topics for the checklist on the following pages were adapted from the results of

ACN's Tic Triggers Survey presented in Chapter 4 and our other data collection efforts. This is not an all-encompassing list, but it is a good place to start. Depending on age and circumstances, a parent should consider discussing possible triggers with a child and asking for feedback, such as whether bright lights cause anxiety or make tics worse, or whether certain foods increase symptoms. Don't be surprised if the child or adult with tics initially denies a reaction to a favorite item, such as video games or sweets, even when he or she knows it makes tics worse. When a child is totally unaware of his or her tics, it is often best to rely on your own observations rather than make the youngster feel self-conscious.

Leaving all options open

If detectives, in trying to solve a mystery, refused to consider certain clues, or decided what the outcome would be before even beginning to investigate, they would not have much chance for success. When making your plans to reduce or prevent symptoms, stay open to all of your options. One of the most common phrases we hear from families is, "Who knew?" when an unexpected benefit occurred from trying a new method.

"Who knew watching television could make my son's tics worse?"

"Who knew mold in the school would cause symptoms to flare?"

"Who knew cutting sugars and milk from her diet would help so much?"

"Who knew scented candles and perfume were irritating my husband's nervous system?"

Sometimes the connections jump right out at you, and you wonder how you ever could have missed them. At other times, the connections were clear only after you kept careful logs over an extended period and reviewed and double-checked your findings.

Later, consider going back through this book for a second reading, focusing on those sections most applicable to you. Take notes, and update them with any new observations. Later, give the "less likely" scenarios a closer look, if needed. (It's where you may find a "Who knew?") You might want to start with relatively easy tasks, adding more challenging ones later. It's possible to develop a list that is so daunting it quickly leads to discouragement.

Keeping your family's sanity—and yours

You will have to balance any passion for "detective work" with a sensitivity to family needs. Motivation can vary widely. Some people would rather experience what they consider a tolerable level of tics than make changes in lifestyle. A sibling or spouse of someone with tics may not feel inspired to make changes (ie, stop wearing perfume, give up having junk food in the house) for the possible benefit of another. At the other end of the spectrum are those who are willing to do "whatever it takes" in search of a complete remission. This range of response is the same as the feedback physicians receive when they recommend changes to patients for weight-loss, diabetes mellitus, heart disease, or other chronic conditions that are impacted by lifestyle.

How to Use the ACN Tic Triggers Checklist

1) Make a copy of the checklist in this chapter (pages 93–95), or download copies from the website: *www.ticsandtourettes.com*.

2) Check-off known trigger items on the checklist now, and add new ones as they are discovered.

3) Be proactive. The checklist is also a "warning" list. You don't have to prove that something is a problem before you eliminate or avoid it. Example: it is known that toxic chemicals, many scented products, and certain types of mold can negatively affect the nervous system. Your entire family will benefit if you reduce exposure to these items. If you happen to find that one or more is a trigger for tic symptoms, then mark it on the Triggers List. (You may wish to circle the boxes next to items when you decide to eliminate them without waiting to observe them as triggers.)

4) Use the Brainstorming Tic Triggers form in Chapter 8 to pinpoint specific factors. Example: if someone has a tic increase after a party, you might wonder whether it was related to a specific food, excitement, an activity during the party, something in the environment, etc. Save the completed sheets to observe patterns.

Family dynamics differ so much that it is impossible to instruct someone on the best method to gain compliance in lifestyle changes without understanding those dynamics. Sometimes the person with tics is thrilled to learn that the symptoms they have might be related to allergies or other issues over which he or she can have some control. Another may react with annoyance or anger at the suggestion that self-discipline is required to start the healing process; it is looked at as just one more burden.

It is important to keep the emotional needs of a child in mind when making changes to diet or activities. Having said that, remember that a youngster does not understand the consequences of poor decisions related to health. It's your job to make responsible decisions for the child.

It is possible to get so involved in reading and scouring the Internet for answers that family members or friends feel neglected and begin to resent the effort. Your dedicated concern may also lead to you feeling overwhelmed, fatigued, or emotionally burned out. When you find yourself in these situations, try to schedule some down time for yourself, and plan family activities where symptoms and efforts to improve health are not discussed.

Reaching out

Many people need professional assistance to reach their goals. Some suggestions for locating help are given in Chapter 22, and the Appendix contains lists of additional practitioner organizations. Keep in mind that the interventions you have been reading about, reported by families, patients, physicians, and researchers, tell us what they found to be most useful. Self-discovery, along with professional guidance, allows you to learn what will be most helpful for you.

A sense of relief

Children may not always want to make adjustments to reduce symptoms, but they usually appreciate when triggers can be found. Learning about causes for symptoms helps them feel more in control. The emotional toll of dealing with unpredictable tics along with accompanying problems like obsessive thoughts can have a dramatic effect on self-esteem. Once triggers start to be identified, the child can begin to think: "It's not me—it's just my allergies!"

ACN Tic Triggers Checklist

These are suggestions for areas to consider as potential tic triggers. It is not a complete list, and not all of these items are relevant to everyone.

A body-mind connection
- ❑ Anxiety, fear, panic
- ❑ Doing nothing (boredom)
- ❑ Listening to someone talk about tics
- ❑ Obsessive thoughts
- ❑ Seeing other people's tics
- ❑ Stress

Classic chemical exposures
- ❑ Chlorine and other swimming pool chemicals
- ❑ Cleaning products
- ❑ Detergents
- ❑ Gas fumes (car, heating, or cooking)
- ❑ Home renovations, new cabinets or furniture, new home
- ❑ New carpeting (toxins)
- ❑ Paint, wood-stain treatments, paint removal products
- ❑ Pesticides (insect treatment, home sprays, bug repellent, freshly treated lawns)
- ❑ Other

Electronics (see also Light)
- ❑ Cell phone use
- ❑ Computer or television use; CRT screen (older, standard cathode ray)
- ❑ Computer or television use; LCD screen (newer, liquid crystal display); or plasma
- ❑ Video games

Food-related
- ❑ Alcohol
- ❑ Artificial colors
- ❑ Artificial flavors
- ❑ Artificial sweeteners

Food-related, continued

- ❑ Caffeine
- ❑ Preservatives and other additives
- ❑ Sweets/sodas/cane sugar
- ❑ Specific foods (Be sure to explore foods eaten three or more times per week in addition to known triggers; use a separate food log, if preferred.)

_____   _____

_____   _____

_____   _____

_____   _____

Infections

- ❑ Viral (flu and cold)
- ❑ Bacterial (strep)

Inhaled allergens (see also Scented products)

- ❑ Dust
- ❑ Grasses, fresh flowers, natural fragrances
- ❑ Mold
- ❑ Pollens
- ❑ Smoke (tobacco, lingering smoke odors, charcoal grill, fireplace)

Light (see also Electronics)

- ❑ Flashing
- ❑ Bright (sunlight, lights at night)
- ❑ Fluorescent
- ❑ Viewing in movie theaters, especially visually intense films

Medications or treatments

- ❑ Allergy or cold medications
- ❑ Stimulant medications
- ❑ Dandruff shampoo to control eczema
- ❑ Other

Movement

- ❑ Car or bus rides (see also Light: and page 262)
- ❑ Changing from a standing or sitting position to a walk or run

Physical—miscellaneous

- ❑ Dental work (braces, spacers, fillings, fluoride)
- ❑ Fatigue
- ❑ Feeling hungry or thirsty
- ❑ Insect bites
- ❑ Vaccines (acute or observable reaction)

Scented products (see also Inhaled allergens)

- ❑ Air fresheners (plug-in type, spray, other forms)
- ❑ Perfume, cologne, or aftershave
- ❑ Typical deodorants
- ❑ Scented candles or artificially scented potpourri
- ❑ Scented personal body soaps, conditioners, and sprays
- ❑ Scented detergent and fabric softeners

Sound

- ❑ Abrupt, loud
- ❑ Background or competing sounds

Temperature

- ❑ Heat
- ❑ Sudden temperature changes in either direction

Touch

- ❑ Clothing and fabric on skin
- ❑ Hand-holding, hugging
- ❑ Heavy touch bothers
- ❑ Light touch bothers
- ❑ Other physical contact

Take away tips for Chapter 7

1) Don't write on your only copy of the ACN Tic Triggers Checklist. You may want to update the information later on a "clean" work page. Blank copies of the checklist are available for downloading from our website: *www.ticsandtourettes.com*. If you don't have access to a computer, we recommend that you make copies of the forms from this chapter before starting to mark down your observations.

2) You should plan to revisit the Checklist occasionally, adjusting your thoughts and findings over time. The Tic Triggers Planner worksheet in Chapter 8 is designed for monthly use. The Brainstorming Tic Triggers form, also in Chapter 8, can be used on an as-needed basis.

3) Stay focused—you can't do everything at once! Select certain areas to investigate based on your situation, and expand your efforts later.

Notes:

_____

_____

_____

_____

_____

_____

8

After the Hunt

ONCE YOU FIND ONE OR MORE TRIGGER SITUATIONS, you will need to begin the process of deciding what to do next. Is the trigger something that can easily come under your control? Does it require a physical change, such as cleaning a dusty bedroom? Does the trigger involve a dietary factor that can be addressed immediately? Focus your attention on each identified trigger, and determine how to best reduce the reaction.

Over time, the immune system can be strengthened through the use of nutritional supplements, detoxification efforts, allergy therapies, or other treatments, along with avoidance of troublesome substances. When this strengthening of the immune system occurs, many of the sensitivities should lessen.

Looking beyond the obvious

When considering a trigger situation, try to uncover all possible reasons why it might cause tics to increase. Do you remember the discussion of the baseball game (page 68)? This is an example of the manner in which you should approach your investigations. Many causes of tic increases will be easy to assess, but at other times some digging and creative thinking will be needed. If you are persistent and ask the right questions, you will be on your way to finding answers. With a little experience it won't be long until you will feel comfortable troubleshooting situations yourself. This comes with practice, however, so be patient. Make a priority list of possible factors, and consider each item on your list, one by one. The Brainstorming Tic Triggers worksheet in this chapter is designed to assist you in this phase of your effort.

If you don't find triggers

This process can take time, especially if you are dealing with a difficult case. If you are not able to locate triggers on your own or you feel overwhelmed, environmental physicians or other practitioners who understand the interaction between the immune system, allergy, toxins, and the brain can often help. They may provide additional medical testing to uncover the cause. (See Chapter 19.) Also, continue to educate yourself by reading the expert advice presented in this book, as well as noting the resources in the Appendix. The website for ACN, *www.Latitudes.org*, and ACN's publication, *Latitudes Online*, can keep you informed of relevant new medical findings (see page 274).

> If you are not able to locate triggers on your own or you feel overwhelmed, environmental physicians or other practitioners who understand the interaction between the immune system, allergy, toxins, and the brain can often help.

It is always possible that you won't find the causes of a symptom, even with some professional assistance. We don't yet know the reasons for this, but two possibilities worth questioning are: (1) whether the approach has been comprehensive enough, and (2) whether you were able to eliminate enough items to separate one triggering event from another.

Additionally, the reaction could involve an issue such as a mild infection that is not causing other observable symptoms and so the possibility for it is not tested. Pediatric autoimmune neuropsychiatric disorders associated with streptococcal infections (PANDAS) is a possibility that may have been overlooked. Perhaps that person has high levels of heavy metals in the body such as mercury, cadmium, or aluminum, that have not been treated. Also, Lyme disease has been known to masquerade as Tourette syndrome and, therefore, may not be diagnosed. Furthermore, a structural problem or state of inflammation could be involved that requires a completely different

Tic Triggers Planner

Name _____ Month _____ Year 20_____

■ **Suspected triggers:**

_____

_____

_____

_____

_____

_____

■ **Goals—triggers to eliminate:**

_____

_____

_____

_____

_____

_____

■ **Observations:**

_____

_____

_____

_____

_____

■ **Notes on progress:**

_____

_____

_____

_____

_____

approach. The possibilities discussed here are not a complete list. In fact, no one yet knows what a complete list would comprise. These are simply examples of the many challenges we face when trying to unravel complex chronic health problems. Just as there are many causes for conditions such as seizures or migraines, there are different reasons why people have tics, and they will not all respond to the same efforts.

Using the Brainstorming Tic Triggers worksheet

When you encounter a situation that results in an increase in tic severity and/or frequency, but you don't know precisely what is behind the increase, use the Brainstorming Tic Triggers worksheet on page 101. Let's take a hypothetical example and assume you are the person with tics. You notice that neck tics developed soon after eating breakfast at home one day. Yet, you aren't sure what specific factor(s) may be responsible.

For "situation" write "Breakfast (date); strong neck tics." Then list all items eaten. Be brand-specific when there are multiple ingredients. Jot the list down while you can remember what you ate; you can check into details later. If anything out of the ordinary occurred that might have played a role in the tics increasing (like an argument at the breakfast table) document that as well, even if you don't think it was related. You are just collecting clues at this point, not making decisions.

For best results, you need to think broadly. Over the coming days, start experimenting with foods and analyzing reactions.

Food—
- Jon's Whole Wheat English Muffin; Butter
- Friendly Farmer's Applesauce (new item tried for the first time)
- Banana

Then list beverages—
- Decaf coffee; cream
- 100% pineapple juice

Supplements at meal—
- Ronna's Multivitamin and Mineral (new item tried for the first time)

Brainstorming Tic Triggers

Date: _____   Describe the situation, including the tic response:

_____

_____

List possible factors:

1. _____   6. _____

2. _____   7. _____

3. _____   8. _____

4. _____   9. _____

5. _____   10. _____

Review your list and develop a game plan for how you can approach this situation to learn more about what may be causing the reaction. List future observations and narrow your list of possible problem factors.

_____

_____

_____

_____

_____

After completing your list, review the items when you have time. If you normally eat that brand of English muffin, check the ingredients to see if new additives have been used. Read the applesauce ingredients; it might contain a lot of regular sweetener, an artificial sweetener, and/or a spice such as cinnamon; each of these can trigger tics in some people. If you normally have applesauce without a problem, this particular brand may be problematic. The multivitamin and mineral that you just started taking is also suspect—it may contain one or more ingredients to which you have a sensitivity. By trial and error you can check each of these possibilities in coming days. You might, for example, decide to try the same breakfast another day without the applesauce. If you don't keep a record, it will be almost impossible to isolate the food items responsible.

Without careful examination, you might incorrectly assume that the reaction you had was due to the breakfast items, when in fact other issues were involved. Eventually you should be able to sort things out, as long as you keep detailed data and ask yourself the right questions. Remember to make photocopies of the blank form, or plan to download them from our site: *www.ticsandtourettes.com*. Be sure to read Chapter 16, on diet, for a more thorough discussion of relevant issues.

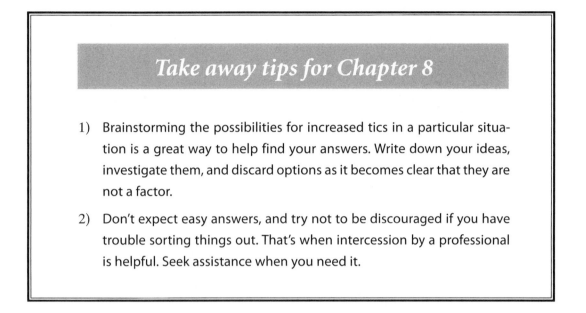

Take away tips for Chapter 8

1) Brainstorming the possibilities for increased tics in a particular situation is a great way to help find your answers. Write down your ideas, investigate them, and discard options as it becomes clear that they are not a factor.

2) Don't expect easy answers, and try not to be discouraged if you have trouble sorting things out. That's when intercession by a professional is helpful. Seek assistance when you need it.

Notes:

_____

_____

_____

_____

_____

_____

_____

_____

SECTION THREE

Sensory Hypersensitivities

CHAPTER

9

Types of Sensory Hypersensitivities

AS INDICATED IN THE SURVEY RESULTS presented in Chapter 4, many people with tic conditions complain of increased sensitivity to one or more of the following: light, movement, touch, odors, sounds, and heat. The phenomenon of sensory hypersensitivity, also referred to as *sensory integrative dysfunction,* is common among learning disabled and autistic populations as well as those with chronic fatigue syndrome and the chemically sensitive.

When you learn to recognize sensory issues that may be aggravating and increasing tic symptoms, you will be in a better position to address those issues. Changes in the environment or treatments to lessen these hypersensitivities can potentially provide relief for more than one type of symptom. For example, when a child is heat sensitive, reducing room temperature and not overdressing the youngster can potentially reduce tics and improve mood if the child is easily aggravated.

All underlying causes of sensory hypersensitivities have not been identified. In addition to the suggestions that follow, the possibility of toxic exposures or heavy metal poisoning (ie, mercury) should be considered when seeking medical solutions. Detoxification or other therapeutic intervention may be needed for a full response. Laboratory testing can determine if there are excess amounts of toxic substances in the body.

Each sensory area is discussed in this chapter, with practical steps for action outlined.

Heat sensitivity

"Mom, it's so hot in here! Put the air conditioning on!" Some children with a tic disorder may be irritable or more symptomatic in warm or hot temperatures, even when those nearby feel fine. They may also start the day comfortably wearing a sweatshirt or jacket, but as soon as they get on the school bus or it begins to warm up outside, they are the first to shed some of their clothes.

As discussed on page 68, results of studies indicate that an increase in room temperature increases tics in approximately one third of adults with Tourette syndrome (TS); some children also struggle with this reaction. Results of the Association for Comprehensive NeuroTherapy's (ACN's) Tic Triggers Survey support this connection; heat was one of the most commonly reported triggers. Similarly, rapid changes in temperature have been anecdotally reported as tic triggers. Family members and friends should be prepared to make adjustments so the child with tics is as comfortable as possible. Here are suggestions for a heat-sensitive child:

> Some children with a tic disorder may be irritable or more symptomatic in warm or hot temperatures, even when those nearby feel fine.

- Try to keep the air temperature as cool as needed to reduce symptoms, even if others need to wear extra clothing;

- Use loose, all-cotton clothing, if that is what feels best;

- Offer a hat for play time outdoors in the sun, and don't overdress a child;

- Make sure cool drinking water is handy when playing outside;

- Initiate fun water activities for children playing outdoors on hot days;

- Buy your child jackets or sweatshirts that are easy to remove;

- Teach your child to self-monitor by learning to watch for signs of heat sensitivity. Encourage your child to communicate needs; and finally

- Consider sensory integration therapy (see page 113).

Touch sensitivity

A hypersensory reaction to touch can aggravate tics. An exaggerated response to touch, known as a *tactile reaction*, can occur when contact is made with other people, furniture, clothing and other items, wind, and food in the mouth. Rough, bumpy, thick, fuzzy, or grainy textures can feel irritating.

Responses to touch may differ. One child might enjoy a light back massage, while such a massage could make another child begin to writhe. If tactile sensitivity seems to be an issue, try the following ideas:

- Cut tags from clothes;

- Wash all new clothes before wearing, and continue washing until soft. Soaking clothes overnight in a laundry tub with a cupful of baking soda, then adding nonallergenic detergent in the wash cycle can help remove some chemicals and odors from new items;

- Wash clothes regularly using a nonallergenic, unscented laundry detergent. Rinse twice;

- Don't force a child to wear clothing that feels irritating. Go for comfort over appearance. Choose all-cotton, loose-fitting clothing;

- Make sure furniture and car upholstery is not irritating. Talk to your child—ask what feels best, and cover with smooth material if needed;

- Avoid ScotchGuard or other chemically treated fabrics;

- Use all-cotton bed linens and blankets; an extra-heavy comforter feels good to some people while others want as little covering as possible;

- Learn what level of touch feels best. If your child avoids being held or touched, it may be due to sensory defensiveness. A firm touch or hug sometimes feels better than a gentle touch or hug—experiment with this; and

- Consider sensory integration therapy, including body brushing, a technique used by therapists to lessen tactile reactions.

Reactions to odors (and chemicals)

Reactions to odors are particularly troublesome to those with chemical sensitivities. Some people with tics also complain of this condition. A heightened sense of smell should alert one or one's family member that low levels of toxic chemicals or other emissions that may not seem to trouble others could be detrimental for this individual. (Of course, not all chemical exposures can be detected by smell.) The following commonsense approaches may help:

- Ventilate the home well;

- Use a vented kitchen fan if food and cooking odors are bothersome;

- Eliminate all scented personal products;

- Don't use scented candles, commercial air fresheners, or scented plug-ins;

- Switch to natural unscented cleansers;

- Don't wear typical perfumes, cologne, or aftershave—and don't allow someone with tics to be exposed to these through others;

- Be responsive to a complaint of an odor, even if you don't notice it;

- Be an advocate for your child at school to be sure that he or she is not being exposed to harmful conditions;

- Avoid new paint and new carpeting, remodeling, new pressed-board furniture and cabinets, and other possible sources of chemical exposures;

- Use a high-quality air purifier with a HEPA filter (high efficiency particulate arrestance). These filters are designed to be more efficient in removing small particles from the air than standard filters; and

- Some odors may be mold-related. Have your home analyzed for mold contamination if you suspect this may be an issue. Mold can have a negative effect on the immune system and has been observed to trigger tics.

Movement

Reports to ACN suggest that the sensation of physical movement itself, such as going from a stationary position to one of action, can cause tics to increase. When a movement problem is associated with motion sickness, explore conventional, homeopathic, or herbal remedies. Also consider possibilities related to movement while riding in a car, bus, or train, and when exposed to moving scenery. (See Chapter 10 on visual sensitivity and page 262 on symptom increases when riding in a car.)

Gerald Erenberg, MD, advised ACN that when tics begin with the anticipation or the onset of physical movement, as when preparing to start running, it may be symptomatic of a rare brain disorder known as *paroxysmal kinesiogenic choreoathetosis*. A movement specialist should be consulted for a proper diagnosis and treatment.

Hypersensitivity to taste (eating or drinking)

When a child refuses a food, it may be because of the taste, the food's temperature or texture, a lack of appetite, fear, swallowing difficulties, stomach upset, or any combination of these. When a child has a developmental delay, or other condition that affects the muscles and chewing/swallowing process, consult a school-based or private practice speech or occupational therapist for advice.

It is obviously important to resolve eating issues because they directly impact health. Some of the following ideas may help:

- Determine whether a hypersensitivity to the feel of foods placed in the mouth is the main issue. Experiment by trying smooth or crunchy foods, or by blending, chopping, freezing, etc, to determine a pattern;

- Introduce a new food to an apprehensive child by allowing him or her to simply lick at it first. Try to determine if he or she is avoiding swallowing or is anxious about swallowing;

- Offer chilled food; this reportedly reduces the taste sensation, compared with a warmer food;

- Understand that nutritional imbalances, digestive difficulties, or swallowing problems could underlie the resistance; and

- Consult with your physician if problems persist.

Auditory sensitivity

Results of the ACN Tic Triggers Survey suggest that large numbers of people with tics are aggravated by sounds. Loud sounds, as well as sudden or punctuating noises—like a sneeze, an alarm or bell going off, or a dog barking, can increase tics in sensitive persons. Constant noises that might not bother others can also be irritating—the hum of a refrigerator or air conditioner, someone talking on the phone while the TV is on, a car engine running, or music playing in the background.

Theories on the cause of sound sensitivity include, in part, a defect in serotonin metabolism, a chemical sensitivity, a deficiency in magnesium and other nutrients, as well as mercury poisoning. Future research should work to define these possibilities. Here are some suggestions for consideration, depending on the particular case:

- Make a concerted effort to minimize noise, once you are aware of hypersensitivity to a sound;

- Try using ear plugs at appropriate times;

- Play some pleasant sounds, such as a CD or a tape of soothing environmental sounds;

- Use a headset with white noise or a masking sound that blocks out the stress-producing noises;

- Consider a trial of magnesium supplementation;

- If problems are not easily resolved, you may wish to look into auditory integration training (AIT). It is sometimes used for autism, ADHD, and learning problems. Although critics contend that proof of its effectiveness is weak, the Autism Research Institute, San Diego, conducted a review of studies on AIT for autism and suggests it can have positive results. Any effort using AIT as a method of reducing tics would be exploratory, as research has not yet been completed in this area.

Sensory integration therapy

Thirty years ago, A. Jean Ayres, PhD, developed a theory of sensory integration dysfunction in children that remains popular. Her therapeutic approach focused on efforts to normalize: (1) sensations of touch; (2) hyper- or hyposensitivity to movement—being overly sensitive to movement or having a lack of appropriate response to movement; and (3) physical feedback and awareness of the body's position in space.

Occupational therapists and others involved with bodywork frequently offer sensory integration therapy. There is controversy over its effectiveness, based on the current research. Yet, many parents, teachers, and therapists insist on its benefits. This may be one of numerous therapies that does not readily lend itself to the standard research model.

Signs of sensory integrative dysfunction, as defined by Sensory Integration International, include *one or more* of the following characteristics:

- Overly sensitive to touch, movement, sights, or sounds;

- Underreactive to sensory stimulation;

- Activity level that is unusually high or unusually low;

- Coordination problems;

- Delays in speech, language, motor skills, or academic achievement; and

- Poor organization of behavior and/or poor self-concept.

If you suspect that your child has a sensory integration disorder, you may wish to seek an evaluation by a qualified physical or occupational therapist.

Visual hypersensitivity

Please see the next chapter for a thorough discussion of the topic of vision and tic symptoms.

Take away tips for Chapter 9

1) Paying attention to sensory situations is a practical and valuable approach you can take when exploring possible triggers. There are many opportunities for environmental adjustments.

2) Your observations, combined with what the person with tics tells you of the experience, will give the clearest picture.

3) Children may not always express what is troubling them. You can help raise their awareness level. Request that they tell you when something like heat, light, a skin sensation, or any of the topics covered in this chapter are aggravating.

4) Be sympathetic and adjust the environment to reduce the sensory triggers when possible.

5) The next chapter highlights vision, a sensory topic that should be considered by everyone dealing with tics.

Notes:

_____

_____

_____

_____

_____

CHAPTER

10

Tics and Visual Sensitivities

A CONNECTION BETWEEN VISION PROBLEMS AND TOURETTE'S has emerged in research during the last 15 years. The studies, small in number yet intriguing, suggest a higher than average number of people with tics experience visual abnormalities. We also know from anecdotal reports to the Association for Comprehensive NeuroTherapy (ACN) that some people with tics are hypersensitive to light, making them more susceptible to light-related triggers that aggravate tic symptoms.

Research suggests that a deficiency in color vision, particularly in distinguishing yellow from blue, can be a common problem with Tourette syndrome (TS) patients. Additionally, according to Jay M. Enoch, OD, PhD, University of California, Berkeley, at least one visual defect is seen in almost all children and adults with TS. Dr. Enoch has suggested that these defects are often related to problems in the field of vision. When we contacted Dr. Enoch, he explained that a visual field test (usually conducted in one eye at a time) assesses the observer's visual sensitivity in different directions, at different locations on the retina. In many of the TS cases he tested, instabilities or changes in visual responses (recorded at the same retinal location across time) occurred. Also, there were characteristic abnormalities in the patterns of visual sensitivity response in the tested eye. Dr. Enoch found that these irregular visual responses could often be traced genetically in a number of modest-size families studied.

Vision problems and toxic exposures

We've just discussed the fact that vision problems often exist among those with TS. Why? What's the connection? Answering this question could bring important answers, but the topic is rarely discussed with families or in the literature for TS.

When reviewing studies for causes of visual defects such as the ones mentioned on the previous page, we learned that color perception abnormalities have been reported following chronic exposure to organic solvents such as *styrene* (a synthetic chemical used in the manufacture of plastics, rubber, and resins); *carbon disulphide* (used in manufacturing cellophane film, rubber and other chemicals); *perchloroethylene* (a hazardous chemical used in dry-cleaning); *n-hexane* and *solvent mixtures* (used to extract vegetable oils from some crops, as cleaning agents, and in glues;) and; *organic and inorganic mercury* (exposures come from seafood, preservatives in vaccines, air pollution, and other sources). Additional vision dysfunctions, such as contrast sensitivity, have also been associated with toxic exposures, mercury in particular. Each of the substances mentioned is also toxic to the nervous system, among other health effects.

We are all exposed to these chemicals at some level through our modern lifestyles. The harmful effect of cumulative exposure to even low levels of numerous toxins has been documented. It seems logical to explore the possibility that toxic exposures may be responsible for both tic disorders and visual deficiencies in some individuals. In the event of identified toxic exposures, detoxification methods should be considered along with strict avoidance of future exposures.

Television and computers: tic culprits

This chapter gives you an overview of visual hypersensitivity, also called *photosensitivity*. We then offer suggestions on ways to explore this possibility and how to help resolve these problems. One of the most common sources of light stimulation is television, so let's start our discussion there.

A large study in 2004 linked television viewing by toddlers and preschoolers with the development of attention deficit hyperactivity disorder (ADHD) at a later age. The more TV that was watched, the greater the chance of an ADHD diagnosis later on. One theory suggests that young brains are being "wired" during the formative years, and TV viewing interferes with optimal brain development. Additionally, time spent in front of a television is time away from normal childhood activities. The possibility of a negative effect of exposure to electromagnetic radiation from the television must also be considered (see next chapter).

> A large study in 2004 linked television viewing by toddlers and preschoolers with the development of ADHD at a later age. The more TV that was watched, the greater the chance of an ADHD diagnosis later on.

No studies on the long-term effects on tics of watching TV exist, but comments to ACN from parents and on Internet forums indicate that tics often increase during TV viewing. The usual explanation for this is that the child is relaxing and feels free to "let the tics out." This concept was reinforced in an article by Samuel H. Zinner, MD, "Tourette syndrome—much more than tics," published in *Contemporary Pediatrics,* August 2004: "Tics usually do not occur during sleep, but are more likely to happen at times and places of personal relaxation, such as while watching television at home." There now appears to be more to the story.

We began looking at this issue more deeply when we heard from a parent named Dawn. Her insight and exploration produced evidence that television viewing itself can exacerbate tics. She discovered that video game play, TV viewing, computer screens, and movies, made her child's tics much worse. Here's Dawn's story:

My daughter's tics started when she was seven years old, and over a period of months, they increased until there were multiple motor tics, sometimes up to four times per minute. Needless to say, my husband and I were greatly concerned. We learned through trial and error that the tics were triggered by the subtle flicker that comes from traditional computer, television, and movie screens. Intense or rapidly flashing images also worsened tics. We are sure now that the problem is a result of visual sensitivity, rather than the excitement or relaxation of viewing because we tested this theory using different situations and types of screens over a period of months.

We found that continued exposure to a flickering screen had a cumulative and lingering effect, meaning it sometimes took several days for the reaction to wear off. Further, the more our daughter was exposed to these screens, the worse her tics became, in number and frequency. We eventually found that an LCD flat screen (liquid crystal display monitor; see pages 120-121) does not have the flicker that a regular TV or computer screen has, and it was not as troublesome.

We first solved the problem by stopping all screen viewing. This allowed my daughter to be completely tic-free! However, she missed having computer and television time. We then bought a 15" LCD computer monitor with a TV tuner. We reduced the monitor brightness for up-close computer work and also had her view TV from several feet away, always in a well-lit room. We further ask her to avoid games that have rapid action or flicker in the image itself. This works for her, and she has no tics when following this plan. She fully understands the situation and cooperates.

I am pleased to report that placing a priority on physical activity, board games, music, and reading over TV and computer time has also improved the quality of our child's life and our family life together. When she needs "down time," music CDs, comic books, and books on tape serve the same function as TV. We are also pursuing integrative medical treatments in an effort to reduce her sensitivity. It has been more than one year with no tics at all.

Once Dawn recognized the role of visual stimuli in tics, she donned the hat of parent-investigator and spent countless hours on our website's forum, convincing other parents to also experiment with reactions to screens. Many were reluctant to deprive their child of their entertainment, but over several months, twenty-two families stepped up to the plate. Twenty of these families saw improvement during a week-long "no screens" test. Longer-term reporting was needed for more meaningful information, so Dawn kept checking in with this group. After two months, although she had lost touch with some of them, 14 families reported that they decided to continue to withhold screen time, either by reducing it or by totally eliminating it (easiest with younger children) because this change helped control the tics. Some also found that LCD screens were a big improvement, and when using them, more time could be allowed on the computer or watching television without a reaction.

To best determine a child's visual sensitivity to screens, Dawn recommends selecting a period when tics are active, and then totally eliminating screen viewing for one week to ten days, both in and outside the home. This includes computers, TV, big screen movies, Gameboys, and even LCD monitors. She suggests that you not start new interventions during this time and that you take note of any other significant triggers that might occur during the testing time that could confuse your findings. Once a clear connection is seen, it is easier to gain cooperation in reducing screen time.

Complete long-term elimination is not an easy task given the amount of time children are accustomed to spending on these activities. However, parents of young children were sometimes successful by stating that there was a "problem with the TV," and it could not be watched. Many parents chose to make a drastic reduction in access to screens, watching carefully for signs of tics when the activity was permitted. As Dawn suggests, trial and error will eventually tell you if this is an issue in your family. Youngsters often respond positively to structured activities and free play in place of television.

What is photosensitivity?

Graham F. Harding, PhD, a professor of clinical neurophysiology at Ashton University in England, is internationally known for his study of seizures and light sensitivity. Dr. Harding wrote an article for *Photosensitive Epilepsy* (1998), and with permission we have adapted some of this material for our discussion. In his article, Dr. Harding explained that photosensitivity is sensitivity to flickering or intermittent light stimulation and/or visual patterns. Such sensitivity causes epilepsy in approximately one in 4000 of the population. In addition, there's an unknown number of photosensitive persons who have not experienced a convulsion but who react negatively to light exposures. It is almost impossible to define this number.

Photosensitivity should be thought of as a *spectrum condition*, ranging from lower levels at which seizures do not occur, to the high end of the spectrum where seizures are easily triggered by light-related factors. Types of seizures that can occur with photosensitivity include *grand mal* (also known as *tonic clonic*), *petit mal* (also termed *absence*), *myoclonic*, and *simple* or *complex partial seizures*. This means that seizures may consist of convulsions, or they may consist of brief episodes of blank staring, rapid blinking or twitching of the mouth or face, jerking movements in other parts of the body, loss of attention, the inability to talk or respond, or sensory hallucination.

For those who are photosensitive, television is the most common source of stimulation, followed by natural and artificial lighting. With television viewing, nearness to the set is a common factor in more than 70% of patients. The flicker rate of the television screen and the content of the broadcast material are also relevant. High contrast, rapidly flashing images can cause seizures or other neurologic responses. Patterns or bars that oscillate (move) are particularly aggravating to vision. Settings that can trigger brain reactions in some people include discos or nightclubs with strobe lights, movies with intense visual images, screens, artificial lighting, and natural lighting. Natural lighting includes such situations as sunlight shimmering off water or flickering through a line of trees.

> For those who are photosensitive, television is the most common source of stimulation, followed by natural and artificial lighting. The flicker rate of the television screen and the content of the broadcast material are also relevant.

Screens and flicker? What to do

A *Latitudes* subscriber who is knowledgeable about the technology involved in the development of television and computer screens sent a helpful letter to improve our understanding of the issues involved in screen flicker:

I have a master of science degree in electronics. I was involved with the television industry for many years and am aware of the differences between the old technology and the current *liquid crystal display* (LCD) technology. My son has a tic disorder. After we switched all our TVs to LCD, he has had fewer symptoms, although they are not completely gone.

When he goes to a friend's home where they have a traditional cathode ray set (CRT) and he plays games on one, the tics increase. This is definitely a factor for some kids, but fortunately this technology is fading away. Although I don't have tics, I am sensitive to the computer monitor's flickering, so I always use high-quality monitors set to the highest possible "refresh" rate, which determines the amount of visual "flicker" on the screen. Check with your monitor manufacturer if you don't know how to adjust this feature. It is often listed as an advanced setting under the monitor display options.

When the refresh rate is set below 70Hz, my eyes become tired, and I develop a headache. It is possible to have a reaction to the flicker, even though you do not "see" it or are not aware of the effect it is having on your brain.

I definitely recommend that anyone dealing with tics or other monitor-related problems switch to LCD or plasma screens. Fortunately, such screens are becoming less expensive. Plasma sets use a special gas, while LCD uses liquid crystals. If you plan to buy one, I recommend an LCD-based set. Plasma technology is newer, and the warranty the manufacturer provides may be shorter than the one provided for LCD.

Other suggestions from vision experts on screen photosensitivity include:

- View in a well-lit room and eliminate reflections on the screen;

- Sit at least 2.5 yards away from a television set and more than one foot back from a computer monitor;

- Wear an eye patch or place a hand over one eye to reduce screen reactions because images must be viewed through both eyes to provoke typical photosensitive reactions;

- Plan to see a movie or attend an event only after checking whether either one has intense flickering or flashing lights, such as strobe lights or visually intense lighting or images.

Additional recommendations include wearing polarized sunglasses outside and avoiding fluorescent lights.

Video games and tics

When parents notice that their child's tics are worse during and after video game play, they often assume, with some logic, that this is due to the stress and excitement of playing the game. However, a vision factor may be involved as well.

Several years ago, widely publicized information from Japan warned that video game use was causing seizures. Since then, warnings have broadened in scope to not only include seizures but involuntary movements, and eye and muscle twitching. It is important to note that you do not need a diagnosis of epilepsy to experience these symptoms. See below:

AN EXCERPT FROM THE NINTENDO® MANUAL (2004) WARNING:

Some people (about 1 in 4000) may have seizures or blackouts triggered by light flashes or patterns, such as while watching TV or playing video games, even if they have never had a seizure before.

Anyone who has had a seizure, loss of awareness, or other symptom linked to an epileptic condition should consult a doctor before playing a video game. Parents should watch when their children play video games. Stop playing and consult a doctor if you or your child have any of the following symptoms (arrows added by editor):

1) *Convulsions;*
2) *Loss of awareness;*
3) *Involuntary movements;* ←
4) *Eye or muscle twitching;* ←
5) *Altered vision; or*
6) *Disorientation.*

To reduce the likelihood of a seizure when playing video games:

1) *Sit or stand as far from the screen as possible;*
2) *Play video games on the smallest available television screen;*
3) *Do not play if you are tired or need sleep;*
4) *Play in a well-lit room; and*
5) *Take a break every 15 minutes.*

"Wearing color" to reduce tics

For the past 20 years, Helen L. Irlen, MS, author of Reading by the Colors *and director of the Irlen Institute, Long Beach, California, has documented visual misperceptions experienced by those with Irlen Syndrome. She discovered the use of color as a treatment to reduce visual hypersensitivity and eliminate perceptual distortions. She shared the following case reviews with ACN, relative to tics:*

Scotopic Sensitivity by Helen Irlen:

Sensitivity to light, learning difficulties, and attention disorders commonly occur alongside the behavioral manifestations of tics. Two cases and their resolution are shared here.

Jessica: Now 19 years of age, Jessica has had frequent eye-blinks, facial grimaces, and throat-clearing throughout her life. Early on, she felt "different" than others, was teased, and had academic difficulties. Jessica found that her tics were worse at school, especially when doing visual tasks. She hated fluorescent lights because they gave her headaches and made her feel tired and anxious. In addition to a diagnosis of TS, Jessica has symptoms of anxiety disorder and attention deficit disorder (ADD). Although she was taking many medications, her problems continued.

Tonya: Tourette syndrome, obsessive-compulsive disorder, and ADD were diagnosed in Tonya at age 19 years. She is now 23 years old. She had poor depth perception, clumsiness, and, at that time, was extremely sensitive to various lighting. Sunlight; glare, even on hazy days; headlights at night; and fluorescent lights made her anxious and gave her headaches. She saw rainbows of colors around things in her environment and around the letters on a white page. Objects in her environment seemed to move rather than appearing stable. Tonya had trouble with concentration and fatigue, and saw herself as anxious. She continues to take Anafranil, Tenex, and Doxeprin, but medication has not helped these symptoms.

For both of these girls, it was their difficulties in school that brought them to the Irlen Institute for a visual evaluation. They knew that sunlight and fluorescent lights bothered them but never connected that annoyance to academic and behavior problems, or tics. During testing, they became aware that they felt uncomfortable and anxious when in rooms with fluorescent lights. Jessica and Tonya realized that visual activities, such as reading, writing, and computer use also caused discomfort and saw that their tics became worse under these conditions. They found a partial solution through a noninvasive technique that we call "wearing color"—using specialized colored lenses or contacts recommended by staff at the Irlen Clinic that can be worn at any time.

> Jessica and Tonya realized that visual activities, such as reading, writing, and computer use also caused discomfort and saw that their tics became worse under these conditions.

Sheets of colored plastic overlays placed on top of pages when reading can also reduce visual stress and symptoms.

The Irlen Method aims to determine the color each individual will wear for the most beneficial results. The exact wavelengths of light, or colors, that are creating the internal stress are identified, and then only those colors are filtered out. Using the wrong color can make problems worse, causing more stress and increased difficulties. Research documents improvement in reading, anxiety, behavior, stress, and headache with the Irlen method. See: *www.irlen.com* to locate Irlen screeners and to review research summaries.

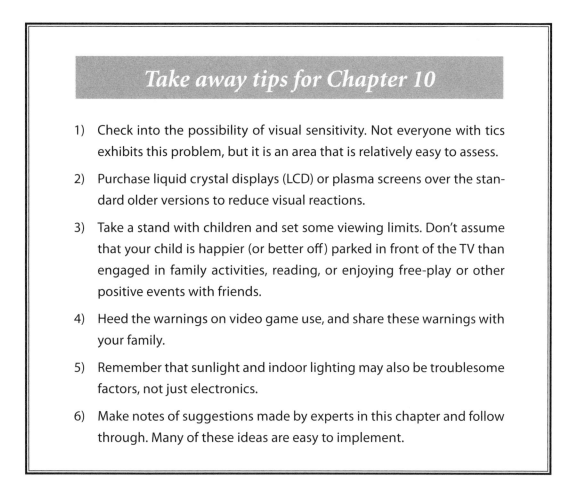

Take away tips for Chapter 10

1) Check into the possibility of visual sensitivity. Not everyone with tics exhibits this problem, but it is an area that is relatively easy to assess.

2) Purchase liquid crystal displays (LCD) or plasma screens over the standard older versions to reduce visual reactions.

3) Take a stand with children and set some viewing limits. Don't assume that your child is happier (or better off) parked in front of the TV than engaged in family activities, reading, or enjoying free-play or other positive events with friends.

4) Heed the warnings on video game use, and share these warnings with your family.

5) Remember that sunlight and indoor lighting may also be troublesome factors, not just electronics.

6) Make notes of suggestions made by experts in this chapter and follow through. Many of these ideas are easy to implement.

Notes:

_____

_____

_____

_____

_____

11

Electrosensitivity and Cell Phones

A COLLEGE STUDENT CONTACTED the Association for Comprehensive NeuroTherapy (ACN) to report that the only time she saw her boyfriend having tics was when he was talking on his cell phone. This report raised a red flag, and we began looking into the issue.

There is concern that increased exposure to electromagnetic fields can aggravate the nervous system. Arthur Firstenberg, director of the Cellular Phone Taskforce, advised ACN that once someone has become sensitized to this radiation, side effects can include tics, headache, nervousness, pain, confusion, and other neurologic symptoms. Firstenberg himself experiences a heightened reaction to electromagnetic radiation, and his health requires avoidance of these fields. Avoidance is an increasingly difficult task because of the proliferation of electromagnetic fields.

Research has confirmed multiple physical reactions to radiation from cell phone stations. Survey responses from a published study in Europe indicated increased complaints of the circulatory system, sleep disturbances, irritability, concentration difficulties, depression, blurred vision, nausea, lack of appetite, headache, and vertigo among those living near cell phone stations. These complaints were made even by those who did not suspect a connection with electromagnetic fields.

To date, no studies have been conducted on electromagnetic radiation and the consequent development of tics. However, Betty Venables, co-coordinator of the Electromagnetic Radiation Safety Network International, informed ACN that her organization occasionally receives reports of adults experiencing neuromuscular reactions or tics when exposed to electromagnetic fields.

A 2004 report confirmed long-standing suspicions that living near overhead power lines increases the risk of leukemia, and a separate study reveals that even extremely-low-frequency electromagnetic fields can be toxic to DNA.

Common sources of electromagnetic radiation include cell phones, cordless phones, computers, televisions, power lines, transformers, security systems, public buildings, lighting, home appliances including microwaves, and cell towers/stations. The issue is highly politicized, with studies that report health concerns met with vehement denials by corporations involved with the booming industries.

Graham/Stetzer Filters have been developed for use in electrical outlets at home or public settings to reduce levels of electromagnetic radiation, termed "dirty power." Research on potential health benefits from use of the filters began recently and remains preliminary at this time. For more information see: *www.stetzerelectric.com.*

> "I have no doubt in my mind that at the present time, the greatest polluting element in the earth's environment is the proliferation of electromagnetic fields. I consider that to be far greater, on a global scale, than warming and the increase in chemical elements in the environment."
>
> —Robert O. Becker, MD

Robert O. Becker, MD, respected author of *The Body Electric,* shared these sobering words during an interview for the Council on Wireless Technology Impacts: "I have no doubt in my mind that at the present time, the greatest polluting element in the earth's environment is the proliferation of electromagnetic fields. I consider that to be far greater, on a global scale, than warming and the increase in chemical elements in the environment."

What the research tells us about cell phones

The use of cell phones is so widespread that we are literally in the midst of a huge global experiment. More than 1,200 medical professionals have signed *The Freiburger Appeal*, initiated in Germany, to express concern about the effects they are seeing in patients that they believe are a result of mobile phone technology. This threat includes not only direct cell phone use but also chronic exposure to cell phone towers.

A review of epidemiologic studies related to possible long-term adverse health effects of mobile phones was completed in 2004. Although all of the studies had some deficiencies, it was concluded that there is an increased risk for *acoustic neuroma* (a benign tumor of the nerve that connects the ear to the brain) and *uveal melanoma* (a malignant cancer of the eye); additional research is needed to confirm this. It is generally assumed that using headsets or speaker phones may help reduce dangers of cell phone use, but this is not yet fully confirmed.

Gro Harlem Brundtland, MD, former Prime Minister of Norway and director-general of the World Health Organization until 2003, has disclosed that she experiences electrosensitivity. Dr. Brundtland did not allow anyone to enter her office at the World Health Organization with a cell phone turned on because, as she explained, an active cell phone gives her a headache. Staff members "tested" this by hiding active cell phones, and the reaction was confirmed. Dr. Brundtland warns parents not to allow their children, whose brains are still developing, to use a cell phone. In 2005, the news media in England carried similar warnings.

> Dr. Gro Harlem Brundtland warns parents not to allow their children, whose brains are still developing, to use a cell phone. In 2005, the news media in England carried similar warnings.

In 2004, it was widely reported that a study by Dr. Imre Fejes revealed sperm count was reduced up to 30% in men who carried a cell phone in stand-by mode on their belt or in a trouser pocket. Although some experts questioned the results of the research, others considered the study to be one more reason to curtail cell phone use. Finally, investigators recently found that mobile phone use may cause headache, extreme irritation, increased carelessness, and forgetfulness.

The ACN has reports from more than 50 people indicating that cell phones aggravate tics. Research on cell phones, though not yet specific to tics, indicates several areas of health concern that suggest a need for careful consideration and expanded study. In the meantime, a cautious approach seems prudent.

Dental work and electromagnetic sensitivity?

We occasionally are informed that dental work has initiated or increased tic symptoms. One case involved a young girl who received metal spacers for her teeth. Her mother reported that after insertion of the spacers, tics immediately started, and they disappeared only months later when the spacers were removed. We don't know whether the metal might have caused an increase in electromagnetic sensitivity with a subsequent nervous system response, whether the appliance put pressure on nerves in the mouth area and this resulted in tics, or whether there is a completely different explanation. On occasion, wearing braces has been anecdotally associated with increased tics, as have new amalgam fillings.

Many factors are involved in dental procedures that might affect tics in sensitive people. A filling with "silver" amalgams is not only a possible conductor for electrical currents, but the mercury used in these amalgams is neurotoxic. A root canal or crown often involves an infection requiring treatments that could further play a role in tic symptoms. A connection between dental work and tics has not yet been adequately explored. ACN is interested in hearing from anyone who has information to share on this topic.

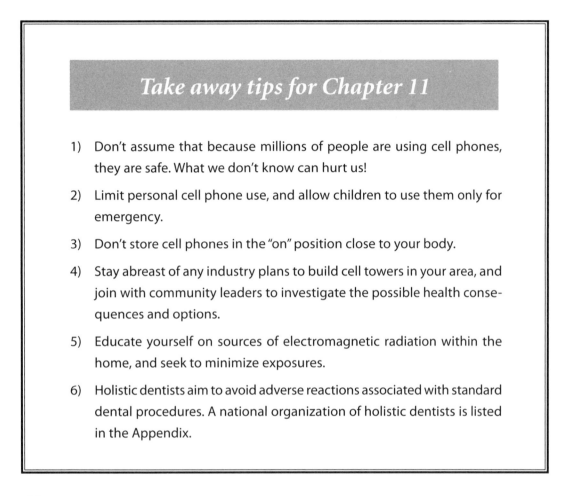

Take away tips for Chapter 11

1) Don't assume that because millions of people are using cell phones, they are safe. What we don't know can hurt us!

2) Limit personal cell phone use, and allow children to use them only for emergency.

3) Don't store cell phones in the "on" position close to your body.

4) Stay abreast of any industry plans to build cell towers in your area, and join with community leaders to investigate the possible health consequences and options.

5) Educate yourself on sources of electromagnetic radiation within the home, and seek to minimize exposures.

6) Holistic dentists aim to avoid adverse reactions associated with standard dental procedures. A national organization of holistic dentists is listed in the Appendix.

Notes:

_____

_____

_____

_____

_____

SECTION FOUR

The Environment and

Immune System Connection

CHAPTER

12

The Critical Environmental Link

WHAT IS HAPPENING TO OUR CHILDREN, and why are nervous system disorders now so common? Possibilities include our changing environment and diet, as well as the standards of treatment to prevent or treat infections and other medical conditions.

Harold E. Buttram, MD, of Woodlands Healing Research Center in Quakertown, Pennsylvania, told ACN: "We are engaged in a battle to save a generation of children from the current trend of deteriorating mental and physical health. Toxic chemicals in the environment, commercial food processing, and overuse of antibiotics are largely responsible for the downward spiral in children's health. It has been estimated that fetuses and children may be ten times more vulnerable than adults to the toxic effects of a class of chemicals known as *volatile organic compounds*. This class includes petrochemicals and a vast number of commercial solvents. The brain and mucous membranes are prime targets. In addition, most children spend excessive hours watching television, using computers, and playing video games. Time spent outdoors in play activities has been greatly reduced."

Dr. Buttram also expressed concern over the large number of vaccines mandated for children, especially those preserved with ethylmercury (thimerosal), which is toxic to the nervous system. In fact, two recent studies suggest a connection between vaccines and tics (see pages 139–40). Once used in almost all vaccines, thimerosal is now being phased out but still remains in some.

School-aged students are taught that the "environment" means the area or world around them. In the medical field, the term takes on an expanded meaning. Environmental factors in medicine include a diverse range of issues, listed below. These issues combine with genetic tendencies to influence health. Even though they have the same genes, the health status of identical twins can differ depending on environmental or experiential factors in their lives such as:

- Food and drink, as well as what one sees, hears, breathes, and touches;
- Stress, fatigue, emotional experiences, and mental states;
- Conditions in the womb;
- Medications and vaccines;
- Infections; and
- Physical impacts (ie, falls, accidents).

This list covers conditions before, during, and after birth. As we have seen from the results of the ACN Tic Triggers Survey (Chapter 4) and letters from families (Chapter 6), many people are aware of the more easily identified factors that may have an effect on their tics.

This section of the book reviews related studies and provides explanations by clinicians that will help you develop a better understanding of why and how the environment and allergies can affect tic symptoms.

Genes as legislator; environment as interpreter

ACN asked medical author, Majid Ali, MD, to comment on the interaction between genetics and the environment for people with tics. He told us, "While tic disorders often run in families, genetic codes are like obscure penal codes—they remain dormant until they are activated by environmental triggers. If this were not so, a hyperactive child would be hyperactive all the time, and a child with Tourette syndrome (TS) would suffer tics all the time. Parents of hyperactive children and those with TS know that it is not so—and so do physicians who care for children afflicted with those disorders."

Let's begin with a look at an early parental report of how the environment significantly affected a youngster's tics. This letter (sent to the Tourette Syndrome Association in the early 1980s) was written by a cardiologist:

> TS was diagnosed in our 15-year-old daughter a couple of years ago. Onset of symptoms occurred at age 11 years. One can imagine our elation in learning there was a medication that would help, and then our disappointment at finding that even on just a minimal dose of the drug, she experienced every side effect in the book, even though her tics decreased by 85%.
>
> We went to Marshall Mandell, MD, an environmental physician. Although my daughter never displayed any typical allergy symptoms, it was found that she is allergic to many foods, some molds and pollens, and is highly sensitive to chemicals. She was placed on a rotation diet (page 186). She has been on the diet for four months and is being desensitized to molds and pollen. I have eliminated as many chemicals as possible from her food and environment. Her reduction in tics while on the diet was 85%.
>
> I took her off the diet while she was on a trip with another family. Within two days, her tics significantly increased, and within one week, they dramatically increased. By dramatic, I mean nonstop tics with several vocalizations, as opposed to one simple tic every one to two minutes, and very slight, if any, vocalizations. Emotional and intellectual patterns that I had not necessarily associated with TS also reappeared at this time.
>
> I observed her reaction to chemicals; with each exposure, her tics would double: An exposure to fluorides doubled her tics for two days; an exposure to a diesel motor running in front of our home increased her tics the entire period the motor ran; an exposure to paint doubled her tics for six hours; an exposure

> "I observed her reaction to chemicals; with each exposure, her tics would double: An exposure to fluorides doubled her tics for two days. . . In my opinion, her sensitivity to chemicals produces a marked increase in the intensity and frequency of her symptoms."

to paraffin in a small restaurant with many burning candles produced nonstop tics until we left the restaurant. In my opinion, her sensitivity to chemicals produces a marked increase in the intensity and frequency of her symptoms.

Had this physician not been vigilant, the sporadic increases in his daughter's tics—which were in fact triggered by foods and chemicals—would have been dismissed as classic examples of the "mysterious waxing and waning of symptoms" described in the medical literature on tic disorders.

Research on environmental triggers for tics

Twenty years have passed since the above letter was written, yet there are few studies that investigate the effect of the environment on tics. A search for additional insight into the role of the environment in tics led to an interesting study involving seasons of the year by Lisa A. Snider, MD, and colleagues. The research focused on 500 children—kindergarten through sixth grade—in Washington, DC. Researchers found that these students had significantly more tics and behavior problems between November and February, compared with levels between March and June. They suggest that an increased tendency to develop infections (eg, strep throat) during the winter months could be an underlying factor in the higher number of tics noted in the period from November through February.

The theory of winter infections leading to increased tics and behavior problems certainly has merit. At ACN, we then brainstormed and took the results a step further, coming up with some additional factors that might be involved in the observed scenario of more symptoms during the winter months:

- In cold weather, children spend most of their time indoors. Hence, they are likely to spend more time playing video games and watching TV than during warmer seasons. This screen viewing and video game use can increase tics in some people (see Chapter 10).

- Depending on the method of heating used, chemically sensitive children could potentially have a reaction to petroleum fuels at school or home that might negatively affect their nervous system.

- Each of the months with high tic rates—November, December, January, and February—are associated with major holidays that are celebrated with artificially colored/flavored candies and other sweets (eg, the "aftermath" of Halloween begins November 1). Many of those working in schools report spikes in discipline problems during the holiday months, from Halloween through Valentine's Day. Research links this type of junk food to behavioral problems, and anecdotal evidence strongly suggests that tics can also be affected by such sugary and additive-laden treats.

- As mentioned earlier, 50% of people with TS are reported to also experience migraine headaches. Researchers have associated migraines and other headaches with weather patterns and changes in barometric pressure. Might the effect of weather patterns themselves play a role in tics? We don't yet know.

Some people see an increase in tics during the spring months, late summer, or early fall, rather than in winter. They often conclude that the increase is a result of exposure to pollen, mold, or other allergens that can be especially problematic at specific times of the year.

Important research linking vaccines and tics

ACN has previously reported on the controversy surrounding the use of the vaccine preservative thimerosal, containing ethylmercury, because of its potential neurotoxic effects. The Institute of Medicine of the National Academies, Washington DC, released a report in May 2004, stating that there is no link between autism or ADHD and vaccines. Some experts have criticized the report as premature and inaccurate. Meanwhile, the preservative is being rapidly phased out of use in most vaccines. Conflicting research is being published, and the topic remains hotly debated and politicized. A new book,

Evidence of Harm, by journalist David Kirby, is a comprehensive and explosive assessment of the way the medical community has addressed this issue.

Results from two recent studies indicate that the use of thimerosal in vaccines has been a cause of tics in children. A large study by Thomas Verstraeten, MD, suggests a link between

> Results from two recent studies indicate that the use of thimerosal in vaccines has been a cause of tics in children.

thimerosal-containing vaccines given to infants and an increased incidence of tics later in life. Additional research in another study in the UK on thimerosal use in the diphtheria-tetanus-whole-cell pertussis or diphtheria-tetanus vaccinations at a young age showed a possible higher risk of tics with the vaccines. Both of these research efforts were retrospective studies (which look back in time after events have taken place, and results are analyzed). If these results indicating an association between vaccines and tics are accurate, they are significant findings with serious implications, yet they have received little attention in the media or by the tic disorders community.

Readers are urged to stay abreast of vaccine issues. Key organizations that promote vaccine safety are listed in the Appendix. Be sure to discuss your options and legal requirements with a knowledgeable health professional.

Environmental medicine: A fundamental contrast

The ACN does not suggest that an environmental approach will benefit everyone with tics. However, for many families, uncovering triggers while treating allergies and strengthening the immune system have been worthwhile efforts. Upcoming chapters in this section of the book contain advice from environmental physicians, each of whom recommends allergy assessment and treatment, dietary management, nutritional therapy, and environmental controls when treating tics. These types of doctors seek to eliminate causes of dysfunction instead of focusing on suppressing symptoms.

In contrast to the diverse backgrounds and training levels of many practitioners who fall under the classic umbrella of "alternative," environmental physicians are fully licensed physicians. These doctors believe they have found a more effective way to treat chronically ill patients than is offered through traditional medicine, and they've adjusted their clinical practices to do so.

There is a divide between conventional physicians and physicians who use nutrition and environmental approaches. One reason for the divide is a difference of opinion on testing and treatment methods, yet it goes deeper than this. Historically, mainstream medicine has downplayed and even resisted recognizing the importance of the environment and nutrition for most neuropsychiatric conditions.

In a book that warns of health consequences for those exposed to toxic air following the attacks on the World Trade Center (entitled *September Eleven, 2005),* medical author Majid Ali, MD, questioned why environmental and nutritional physicians are rebuffed by many in the medical community. He also asks in a rhetorical manner why these professionals stick with their newly found professional path when they could make more money much more quickly, by simply relying on a prescription pad. He suggests:

"We [environmental and integrative physicians] are all prisoners of the truth. Truth that sick people can get well without drugs, truth that nutrients facilitate that process, truth that drugs do not solve the underlying chronic problems of health, truth that drugs work by blocking the very enzymes and mediators that we need for healing, truth that as necessary as drugs are for acute life-threatening illness, the concept that drugs can promote health is fundamentally a flawed concept. Once we know this truth, we cannot back away from it. We are captives of the truth—prisoners of truth."

Tics as an immune response to environmental factors

Marshall Mandell, MD, was the first physician to systematically record tic responses to allergenic substances for numerous patients with TS. A best-selling medical writer in the field of environmental medicine, Dr. Mandell took a special interest in tics and Tourette syndrome in the early 1980s. He recruited patients with TS and evaluated and treated them at his own expense. The results convinced Dr. Mandell of a critical connection between the environment, diet, allergy, and tics. He explained:

> I saw 26 TS patients over the course of several months. I used a single-blind method of testing in which the item for which the patient was being tested was unknown to the patients and parents. I found that for approximately 80% of these individuals, their typical patient-specific TS symptoms were

aggravated by allergenic extracts of chemical agents, airborne allergens, and foods. I found that allergy treatment, dietary and environmental changes, and nutrient supplements could help most, though not all, TS cases seen.

Around this time, Dr. Theron Randolph (see page 260) told me of a seven-year-old boy with a moderately-severe case of TS who came under his care. The boy's medications were discontinued, and he was evaluated by Dr. Randolph as part of an in-hospital program of comprehensive environmental control. This program consisted of fasting on spring water in an uncontaminated environment. The boy's tics and vocalizations completely disappeared on the fifth day of this spring-water fast. After these symptoms cleared, the boy had a series of single-food test meals ("challenges" with organically produced foods). Each meal consisted of a generous serving of one of the foods he usually ate—without spices or sauces. The only seasoning permitted was untreated sea salt. This method accurately identified the dietary factors causing symptoms of TS, as certain items brought on episodes of his symptoms. He was discharged, symptom-free, after his dietary offenders had been identified. Dr. Randolph's only "prescription" for this patient was a diversified rotation diet with tolerated foods that did not cause TS symptoms.

> The fact that this remission occurred at all should be of interest to clinicians who consider TS symptoms intractable without drugs. A cause-and-effect relationship between eating specific foods and the appearance of this patients' symptoms was clearly demonstrated.

I am not advocating fasting or suggesting that all individuals with TS would respond in this manner, but the fact that this remission occurred at all should be of interest to clinicians who consider TS symptoms intractable without drugs. A cause-and-effect relationship between eating specific foods and the appearance of this patients' symptoms was clearly demonstrated. I have been in touch with other physicians whose patients with tics similarly improved with nutritional and immune approaches.

Later, I pursued triple-blind tests in which the patients were put on rotary diversified diets before the double-blind codes were broken and no one knew which food test would be expected to cause familiar symptoms. This test had positive results, confirming that tics were exacerbated by eating certain foods.

In addition to the effects of food culprits, a patient may also be an undiagnosed "chemical reactor," that is, a chemically susceptible person who reacts to tic-provoking chemical agents that are inhaled, ingested, or absorbed through the skin. To further complicate matters, some individuals have brain sensitivities to various inhaled allergens like dust mites; molds; tree, grass and weed pollens; animal danders; bacteria; and viruses.

Shortly after this discovery, I attended an International Scientific Symposium on Tourette Syndrome sponsored by the Tourette Syndrome Association. There, I listened to numerous reports of drug therapies for TS and concerns about their side effects on patients. Recognizing the importance of my discovery, I went to the front of the room and informed all the researchers and physicians in attendance of my findings. I explained that they could help their patients by learning more about the role of the immune system in TS, and that by having patients address environmental issues in their lives, they could reduce their dependence on medications. To my profound disappointment and surprise, *not one person there* expressed any interest, asked a single question, or followed up on my findings.

I predict that nutritional, allergic, and immune factors will be found to be key factors in the development of tics. Unfortunately, by that time, thousands of families will have suffered needlessly.

Editor: Dr. Mandell's conclusion made 20 years ago was correct, and, even today, it is still not recognized by mainstream medicine. We salute him for his selfless and insightful pioneering efforts. His reports were soon followed by similar accounts from Doris J. Rapp, MD, who linked symptoms of TS to allergy in her best-selling book, *Is This Your Child?*

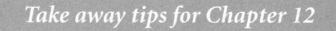

Take away tips for Chapter 12

1) Don't wait for studies to tell you if something within your control may be affecting your child. Look into it yourself. Published research on environmental issues that affect tics is very limited.

2) Make healthy choices. Decisions you make every day can affect your family.

3) If you are a prospective parent, follow through on prenatal wellness advice from your doctor, and avoid exposure to neurotoxic chemicals.

4) Make educated decisions on vaccinations and discuss the topic with your physician. Read labels on vaccine vials to be sure they do not contain thimerosal.

Notes:

_____

_____

_____

_____

_____

_____

_____

13

Tics and Modern Lifestyles

Joseph S. Wojcik, MD

The author of this chapter, Joseph S. Wojcik, MD, is board-certified in allergy, asthma, and sinusitis in infants, children, and adults. He is a practicing physician in Bronxville, New York. Dr. Wojcik is a fellow of the American College of Allergy, Asthma, and Immunology and a fellow of the American Academy of Environmental Medicine.

ALTHOUGH THE BASIC CAUSES OF CLASSIC TIC DISORDERS, including Tourette syndrome, are still unknown, current research propounds an abnormality in the genes affecting the brain's metabolism of the neurotransmitters dopamine, serotonin, and norepinephrine. The enigma remains: What triggers the neurotransmitters to evoke the tics?

An escalation in gene abnormality

The surge of tic disorders in recent years did not suddenly appear per chance, for no reason. I believe an answer to the epidemic of tics, cancer, autoimmune diseases, metabolic diseases and the like is obvious. It relates to Nobel Prize winner Barbara McClintock's premise of *jumping genes*, that suggests that the genes with which you were born can change under particular circumstances. McClintock's findings have wide implications and help us understand how the stressors in our modern lifestyles can modify the genome. In other words, we don't all continue to have the same genes we were born with—and the same is true for our parents!

The cause of gene modifications

There is one obvious answer to why genes are being rapidly modified. We have simply been in denial and have ignored the staggering mountain of data clearly staring us in the face. Marketers in the 20th century did a monumental job of seducing the public to believe in and adapt a new, modern lifestyle, a "better way of living." The public was offered relief from the time-consuming "drudge" of cooking and the pain of doing dishes. Foods were now available, fully cooked and ready to eat in minutes, with beverages of all varieties.

Processed foods of all shapes, sizes, and colors were delivered to the public in delectable, enticing packages. Vitamins, minerals, amino acids, essential fatty acids, and other essential nutrients were deliberately removed during processing to extend their shelf life. Plastic foods had arrived.

Our bodies are constantly undergoing catabolic and anabolic recovery (metabolic breakdown and synthesis). These processes require a constant infusion of nutrients that come primarily from our diet, and secondarily from supplements, for those who take them. Over time, abnormal changes occur within our organs, and eventually, our bodies begin to exhibit symptoms. Some metabolic systems shut down, and others react inappropriately. The biochemical makeup that took millions of years to develop is trashed by this constant abuse occurring over relatively few years. As our organs and tissues did not know how to react to this ongoing abrogation of the norm, they responded abnormally with tics, autoimmune diseases, and a multitude of other "new" diseases.

My experience with tics and Tourette syndrome

I practiced pediatrics for 25 years before becoming board-certified in allergy and environmental medicine. Tics were not an uncommon finding in young children and even adults, most commonly as eye-blinking and facial tics. However, they usually spontaneously cleared after several months. Despite my reassurances that they were benign and would abate as readily as they had appeared, parents remained concerned until that joyous moment when the tics were gone. However, in the past 15 years, there seems to be an "epidemic" of patients with multiple tics, particularly classic Tourette syndrome (TS).

My initial exposure to TS occurred approximately 25 years ago. I had been pediatrician to two brothers for several years. Their general health was always normal with the exception of occasional respiratory infections.

During an office visit, one of the brothers presented with TS symptoms including facial tics, eye-blinking, neck-snapping, shoulder-shrugging, jumping, touching, sniffling, and throat-clearing. He was an intelligent teenager with an above average academic profile and had no coexisting syndromes or illnesses. His developmental milestones had always been within normal parameters. A comprehensive history suggested food allergies, pollen allergies, and mold allergies. This was documented by a dietary elimination and challenge diet, as well as by RAST (*radioallergosorbent test*) evaluation. The boy's TS symptoms lessened significantly after he started immunotherapy for food and inhalant allergies and even further with diet modification, nutritional support, and use of biofeedback. He was delighted that he was able to become his own personal detective, and he immediately began investigating which foods triggered tics. Once discovered, he avoided those foods, except for those he craved or was addicted to, and he ate those only when his craving became overwhelming.

Environmental measures, such as cleaning his cluttered bedroom, removing old, musty carpets, and other allergy control efforts helped contain the frequency of his symptoms. Over time, he became more self-assured, happier with himself, and happier generally. The tics continued to resolve.

Since that time, I have seen a number of similar cases that have responded to these approaches, although each has its own profile.

A PANDAS patient responds to immunotherapy

My most recent patient, Tom, proved to be a case of PANDAS (pediatric autoimmune neuropsychiatric disorders associated with streptococcal infections; pages 13–15) with symptoms similar to Tourette syndrome. His tics started when he was nearly four years old, following a strep throat. Over the next few years, Tom had four more strep throats, and, predictably, his symptoms flared with each infection. Although the symptoms lessened after treatment with antibiotics, they remained problematic.

Tom's parents were extremely keen on cooperating because their son's tics were severe. His tics included a twitchy face, eye-blinking, neck-snapping, arm-twisting, leg-jerking, sniffling, throat-clearing, barking, self-inflicted wounding, poor concentration, and echolalia (repeating others' words).

Tom's parents revised his diet and cleaned up a mold problem in the home, and 80% of the tics dramatically cleared. The parents were ecstatic at the rapid change, although with time, they permitted him to cheat and to eat foods he craved because "he had been such a good boy." Of course, some tics would then resurface. His parents now know that the symptoms generally clear within four days—the normal time required for clearance of most foods from the gut—so they are not overly concerned when this happens. This is not a good situation to encourage, however, because when Tom becomes a teenager and has money in his pocket, he may not be able to control his cravings and his tics may not so readily go away.

Finding a standard approach for tic disorders

In my experience, there is no standard protocol for tic disorders. Each patient is individual because each has his or her own biochemical profile. During review of a comprehensive questionnaire or food symptom journal, it often becomes obvious to the parents or adult patient that the tics are directly aggravated by foods and environmental exposures. Testing further confirms this idea. Of course, allergies to molds, pollens, and other allergens that may also trigger tics have to be tested and treated. Parental and child cooperation in following through on recommendations is key to a successful response.

The biggest hurdle: Food cravings

The greatest obstacle for most parents and patients to surmount is eliminating foods they crave that obviously trigger symptoms. Often, patients with tics are virtually addicted to certain foods. Eliminating these foods presents as great a challenge to the "food addicts" as eliminating the addictions of smokers, alcoholics, and drug users. The patient needs treatment that includes behavior modification, dietary modification, and constant encouragement to overcome addiction to these foods.

What is often not recognized is that one or both parents may be addicted to the same foods as the child and may continue purchasing the food for their own consumption, to satisfy their own cravings. Telling a child not to eat a food to which they are addicted is easy. Getting cooperation when the pantry is not "squeaky clean" is impossible.

In summation, our protocol for treatment of tic disorders uses diet modification; allergy immunotherapy; cleaning up the home, school, and work environments; faithful taking of recommended supplements; and following through on biofeedback if indicated, along with any other prescribed measures.

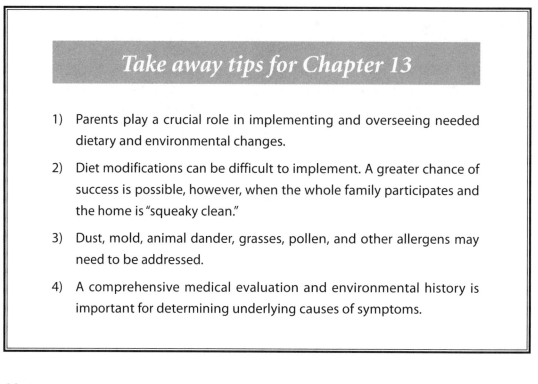

Take away tips for Chapter 13

1) Parents play a crucial role in implementing and overseeing needed dietary and environmental changes.

2) Diet modifications can be difficult to implement. A greater chance of success is possible, however, when the whole family participates and the home is "squeaky clean."

3) Dust, mold, animal dander, grasses, pollen, and other allergens may need to be addressed.

4) A comprehensive medical evaluation and environmental history is important for determining underlying causes of symptoms.

Notes:

_____

_____

_____

_____

_____

_____

_____

14

Why Sherlock Holmes Would Be Shocked

An Interview with Dr. Albert Robbins

In this interview, Albert E. Robbins, DO, MSPH, discusses principles that can be helpful for understanding the role of the environment, diet, and nutrition in tic disorders. Dr. Robbins is board-certified in both preventive medicine, and occupational and environmental medicine. He is a fellow of the American Academy of Environmental Medicine, a Diplomate of the international and American boards of environmental medicine, and former editor of the Environmental Physician. (Interview by Sheila J. Rogers.)

Dr. Robbins, I know you have a special interest in tic conditions. How did that interest develop?

It was serendipitous. While treating patients for allergy, we found that some who also had tic disorders (including Tourette syndrome), hyperactivity, and/or obsessive-compulsive disorder, reported symptom relief, not only from their traditional allergies, but also for these neurologically related symptoms. I began to explore this angle more comprehensively. And we later had the dramatic case of Griff Wakem, whose severe symptoms improved so remarkably with this approach.

I've treated more than 100 allergic patients who also had one or more of these overlapping central nervous system disorders and have found each case to be challenging and unique. Although we cannot help all patients with tics or Tourette's, we can identify some of the environmental or allergic triggers that such patients attribute to the waxing and waning of their condition.

I should mention that I am not the first to observe this environmental/neurologic connection. Theron G. Randolph, MD, the "father" of environmental medicine, Marshall Mandell, MD, and Doris J. Rapp, MD, all reported an environmental connection for tics and TS more than 18 years ago. Further, there are many other physicians who are successfully using an environmental approach for these central nervous system disorders. This is an observational approach to a neurologic disorder that appears to have allergic triggers.

What do you mean by an environmental or observational approach?

This approach uses a Sherlock Holmes-type of investigation that searches for environmental clues to the triggers that either cause or aggravate disease. These clues comprise both internal and external susceptibility factors that may modify disease states and include everything we eat and drink, breathe, and use. Certainly, this would include stress factors, diet, personal care products, geography, climate, seasonal variations, infections, exposures to chemicals, allergens, pets, biologic agents (parasites), and other reservoirs of disease. Common environmental allergens include pollens, dusts, molds, animal danders, and certain foods. After the investigation is complete, we then create a treatment plan that includes avoidance (environmental controls) and allergy desensitization.

Exposures to certain common chemicals are known to produce serious neurologic effects in susceptible individuals. Such chemicals include perfumes, pesticides, and *volatile organic compounds* (VOCs), such as formaldehyde, fabric softeners, naphthalenes or mothballs, and phenols, such as those found in Lysol cleanser. Air fresheners (both aerosol and plug-ins) may contain p-dichlorobenzene. New carpeting also contains offgassing chemicals. Moldy homes and offices can release VOCs that give the air a musty odor and can affect the nervous system. Finally, I should also mention cigarette smoke as a serious offender.

Many chemical products, particularly when used indoors, make the environment dangerous for the environmentally hypersensitive—those with allergic disease, asthma, and chemical hypersensitivities. Patients with tics, therefore, would be wise to avoid exposures to indoor chemical agents; they may test this hypothesis for themselves. My experience has been that some patients have a marked decrease in symptomatology when they avoid these agents completely.

Control of inhalants including mold is also important. Mold has been associated with periodic limb movement disorders in published research. There are reports that people exposed to mold from water damage in buildings found an increased risk of autoimmune response, such as inflammation, as well as neurologic reactions affecting the central and peripheral nervous system.

I understand you're an osteopathic physician, board-certified in preventive medicine, with a subspecialty in occupational/environmental medicine. Could you explain for our readers what an osteopathic physician is?

In the United States, an osteopathic physician, or DO, is equal to an allopathic physician, or MD, in medical education, licensing, right to hospital affiliation, board-certifications, and medical specialties. Osteopathic physicians practice medicine in all states throughout the country, under equal status as MDs. The only major difference is that osteopathic physicians have received training in manipulation—which they may or may not use in their practice—and they are trained to approach health and illness from a more holistic orientation than MDs. By holistic orientation, I mean looking more at lifestyle factors whenever possible as contributors to health and illness, rather than just prescribing medication.

For example, for decades I've advised patients with hypertension to follow a diet that's high in fruits, vegetables, and fiber and low in saturated fat, and salt, and instructed them also to exercise regularly. Just recently, results of studies have confirmed that this approach can be used as an initial therapy for the treatment of mild hypertension and may work as well as medication in some cases. An environmental approach that examines lifestyle issues for people with tics also promises to be helpful.

Is environmental medicine expensive?

Cost is always a factor when considering medical treatments. I suggest that families educate themselves in principles of environmental medicine and test the environmental principles for themselves. Before the initial office evaluation, I usually recommend avoidance of certain foods, allergens, and chemical exposures. If they find a connection between symptoms and exposure during the trial period, then assessment and treatment is usually warranted.

Parents and children have told me that their symptoms improve when they avoid certain common foods and scented personal care products. We ask patients to keep a diary of when and where symptoms are better or worse in an attempt to isolate environmental factors. This tracking includes the effect of foods, chemicals, and indoor environments. Such assessment and treatment is relatively brief and inexpensive.

When further evaluation is required, comprehensive allergy skin testing, laboratory blood tests, stool evaluations, urine and hair testing may be recommended. Allergy vaccines, routine office visits, and environmental changes may certainly be worth the expense. However, it would be prudent to begin a trial of environmental allergy and chemical avoidance along with an allergy elimination diet first. It is not wise to spend a considerable amount of money on testing and treatment without understanding the underlying environmental principles involved. One must work within the boundaries of science and utilize environmental principles appropriately to improve chances for good results.

Does research support the allergy connection to Tourette syndrome?

One of the most significant articles related to allergies and Tourette syndrome was reported several years ago in the *Journal of the American Medical Association*. The authors reported on identical twins, detailing a relationship between TS symptoms and environmental factors. The authors observed that although the twins had an identical genetic makeup, their TS manifested differently in each, with varying degrees of severity. I recall also that the authors suggested "optimizing the environment" to lessen the impact of the genetic predisposition but specific suggestions were not given. I believe that a thorough environmental medical approach is an appropriate place to start.

There are also cases of TS in which we see no family history of the disorder, clearly emphasizing the importance of looking thoroughly at environmental factors, including allergy.

Another example of movement disorders being triggered by foods, or components in food comes from a published report from the College of Medicine at the University of Saskatchewan. In the study, one person reacted with increased movement when exposed to milk, another had a similar reaction to coffee and eggs, and a third to aspartame (NutraSweet). Considerable literature regarding multiple allergies supports the concept of brain or neurologic allergy. Jonathan Brostoff's comprehensive textbook entitled *Food Allergy and Intolerance* frequently mentions food and chemical factors as triggers of multisystem allergic disease, including neurologic symptoms. Frederick Speer's textbook, *Handbook of Clinical Allergy* includes a chapter entitled "Neurological Allergy." In addition, Speer authored a textbook on the subject, entitled *Allergy of the Nervous System*. Brennan's classic textbook, *Basics of Food Allergy*, also makes reference to certain foods triggering allergic reactions in the brain and affecting behavior. Other references include Houston King's textbook, *Otolaryngic Allergy*, and Joseph Miller's book, *Relief At Last*. Both of these texts include discussions of neurologic symptoms as possible manifestations of allergic disease.

Many neurologic aspects of multiple chemical sensitivity are discussed in William Rea's four-volume classic, *Chemical Sensitivity*. Neurologic symptoms of chemical sensitivity can include dizziness, tremor, fatigue, hyperirritability, tics, headache, spaciness, muscle spasms, and even hypersexuality.

The environmental connection to tic disorders has not yet been formally researched. Such research needs to be undertaken now as recent studies indicate that individuals with TS have a higher level of classic allergy than the general population.

What do you mean when you refer to testing these principles?

First, families need to understand that someone can have a genetic predisposition to TS, but controlling his or her environment can make a significant difference in how that predisposition plays itself out. For example, someone may have a tendency toward dust allergy, but if he or she has an allergen-free home, there may be few symptoms. Another person having a similar predisposition could live in a very dusty home and struggle with significant allergic symptoms.

The concept is simple, but following through on a comprehensive environmental plan takes self-education, discipline, and some effort. I typically ask the family to replace smelly chemical products with safer, hypoallergenic, fragrance-free ones. I also suggest making the home as allergen-free as possible and initiating a trial allergen elimination diet. In addition, the family should eliminate any foods or environmental agents that are suspected of triggering or aggravating tics or any other annoying symptoms.

I was asked to speak at a TS support group, and you may be interested in some of the comments. They asked for dietary recommendations, and after discussing that, we began talking about other environmental issues. One mother, who was concerned about her young son's Tourette's, told us that her home is filled with scented candles, potpourri, and other fragrances. I recommended that she eliminate all of these, pointing out that this action might help her son and might also help relieve her migraine headaches. They also had a cat, and I suggested that she at least keep the cat out of her son's bedroom and have her son tested for cat allergy. If he proved allergic to the cat, they then should consider having the cat live elsewhere.

A father remarked that he had recently had their home sprayed for bugs and had noted a dramatic increase in his son's tics around that time. He asked whether there was a chemical connection to his tics. He also described observing his son calmly doing his homework, seemingly very focused. The boy then ate a candy bar. Within minutes he was overly active, had more tics, and could hardly concentrate on his work. This type of observation can confirm a food connection. Perhaps these individuals are simply more hypersensitive to a wider number of environmental factors than the rest of us.

Usually a complex constellation of factors—including biologic problems—are the true triggers of the reaction that results in tics. Obviously, everyone exposed to the same environmental conditions does not have the same experience.

Do you think all people with Tourette syndrome have an allergy connection?

Tourette syndrome is a complex condition with as yet undefined genetic and environmental variables. Although many people with tic disorders, including TS, have reported moderate to dramatic improvement with the approach we use, not everyone has benefited. We don't yet know which subgroups of individuals are most likely to respond positively, yet in my experience, individuals with common allergic symptoms, including nasal allergies and asthma, appear to benefit most.

Our modern lifestyle has led to an increase in allergic disease. Pesticides were developed more than 60 years ago when the chemical industry was in its infancy. The increased use of chemical products over our lifetime may play a significant role in the production of allergic and numerous neurologic diseases. This issue needs further exploration.

You previously mentioned infection as an environmental factor. What does infection have to do with central nervous system symptoms?

Infection causes the body to attempt to defend itself. The body produces immuno-logic factors that communicate with the rest of the body. One of those communication networks is within the nervous system. There is a recognized neuroimmune connection in the body. The body functions as a unit, and if any portion of any biologic system is affected, that dysfunction can affect other areas of the body as well. A hidden infection can cause multiple secondary biologic problems. Therefore, it's important to rule out infection as a factor in all tic conditions. Strep infection has been mentioned as a possible trigger. There may be others including viral, bacterial, fungal, or parasitic organisms.

What are the nutrients you most often recommend?

I can give some general guidelines. Some nutrients are considered helpful by many authorities for improving immunologic and neurologic function. For example, Abram Hoffer, MD, an orthomolecular psychiatrist, found that various forms of vitamin B_3 have been used successfully in treating some forms of schizophrenia. Taurine is an amino acid that has calming and antiseizure effects on the nervous system. Zinc and vitamin B_6 when taken together have been shown by some investigators to improve immunologic and neurologic function. Calcium and magnesium are sometimes used for better muscle and nerve function. Vitamin B_{12} and folic acid are useful for various neurologic and digestive disorders. Some physicians use pantothenic acid (vitamin B_5) for stress disorders, as B_5

supports adrenal function. Vitamins B_1 and B_2 are important to calm the nerves. Finally, essential fatty acid supplementation may be beneficial.

However, for more accurate and appropriate nutritional intervention, a physical examination and nutritional blood tests are necessary to detect vitamin and mineral deficiencies and to identify possible amino acid metabolism disorders. In addition, hair analysis and urinalysis are sometimes used to diagnose heavy metal toxicity (ie, lead, mercury, copper).

What about heavy metals?

I often look for elevated mercury, lead, and copper concentrations, as well as deficiencies in magnesium and zinc. Levels of other toxic metals can also be assessed. These metals have often been associated with neurologic dysfunction. It's important to determine whether a mineral imbalance is serious and clinically significant. For example, it has been established in the literature that there is a relationship between zinc and copper. High copper levels and low zinc levels are associated with hyperirritability of the nervous system. When you increase the amount of zinc, you drive the copper levels down because of their reciprocal relationship in the body.

Chelation therapy through the use of oral dimercaptosuccinic acid (DMSA), for example, has been an accepted treatment for the removal of heavy metals, particularly lead, for decades. Other agents are also used. Chelation therapy should be closely supervised, and particular care taken when working with children. If one finds serious heavy mercury or lead toxicity, I recommend that chelation therapy be pursued in consultation with a knowledgeable neurologist or toxicologist.

Readers relate that their neurologists often tell them they are wasting their time in pursuing dietary changes or nutritional therapy.

Neurologists should not be hesitant to refer patients with tics for an environmental/allergy investigation. They should also recommend healthful lifestyles, which include regular physical exercise and nutrient-rich diets. Further, nutritional evaluations and testing, along with immune studies, should be emphasized in the workup of all TS patients.

I find that families are usually aware that stress and emotional factors aggravate tics, but they are not generally aware that the patient may be a victim of unknown environmental factors. An environmental allergy approach certainly poses less of a risk of side effects than the prolonged use of many drugs. If you are a parent dealing with TS, you won't want to overlook the opportunity of exploring this environmental approach. The evaluation and treatment of TS does not belong exclusively to the domain of psychiatrists and neurologists. Immunologists, allergists, environmentalists, and nutritionists may be able to make a difference in treatment outcomes.

Why do you emphasize avoidance of scented products and certain chemicals?

The brain is rich in special enzymes, acetylcholinesterases, and chemicals, such as serotonin, dopamine, and others, that govern the triggering and firing of nerves. *Organophosphate pesticides* as well as VOCs, such as perfumes and formaldehyde, can alter the release of some of these brain chemicals. Changes in brain chemistry can alter neurologic function. Some individuals have a hypersensitivity or allergy that affects these brain chemicals, causing a neurotransmitter chemical imbalance.

Why is there so much controversy in the medical community over the concept of multiple chemical sensitivity?

Physicians know very well that various chemicals can adversely affect many biologic systems, including the nervous system. One main issue has been accepting the fact that low levels of these same chemicals can have a significant effect in hypersensitive persons. Many physicians are fearful of making a diagnosis of multiple chemical sensitivity (MCS)—though they are clearly seeing these patients in their offices. Very few physicians fully understand the significance and severity of the MCS problem and its impact on a wide number of chronic illnesses. It is a difficult concept to understand unless one actually has the problem.

Anyone wanting to know more about MCS can refer to Ashford and Miller's textbook, *Chemical Exposures, Low Levels and High Stakes*, second edition. This book discusses the medical controversy surrounding MCS.

It seems food allergy treatment also stirs up controversy.

Some physicians do not believe in food allergy treatment. The controversy has to do with the types of food allergy tests and types of treatment that are used today. Some forms of allergy testing and treatment are controversial, and some types of testing are not reproducible.

When patients are sensitive to a wide number of foods, they are usually also sensitive to chemicals. There is a food-chemical interaction. When we treat them for their food allergies and desensitize them, they are often then better able to tolerate foods and also they tend to react less to some chemicals. Similarly, there is also a cross-desensitization with certain pollens and foods. For example, if one is allergic to ragweed, there may be a concomitant reaction to milk, melon, and bananas. Also, if one is mold-sensitive, one should avoid mold-related foods, such as cheese, mushrooms, honey, fermented and pickled foods, as well as foods containing yeasts and sugars.

Tics can be triggered by any number of factors. I must say, Sherlock Holmes would be surprised that the Tourette community has missed the environmental clues!

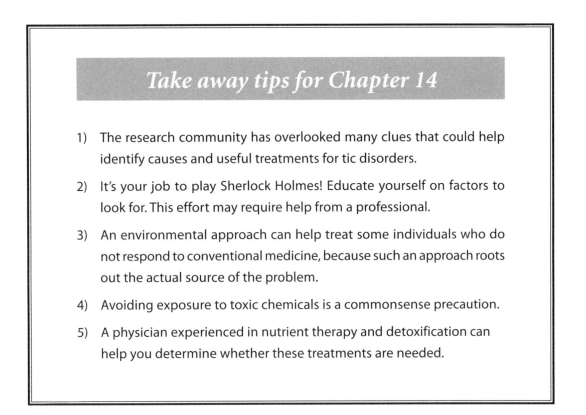

Take away tips for Chapter 14

1) The research community has overlooked many clues that could help identify causes and useful treatments for tic disorders.

2) It's your job to play Sherlock Holmes! Educate yourself on factors to look for. This effort may require help from a professional.

3) An environmental approach can help treat some individuals who do not respond to conventional medicine, because such an approach roots out the actual source of the problem.

4) Avoiding exposure to toxic chemicals is a commonsense precaution.

5) A physician experienced in nutrient therapy and detoxification can help you determine whether these treatments are needed.

Notes:

_____

_____

_____

_____

_____

_____

15

Autoimmunity in Brain Disorders and Mental Illnesses

Vijendra K. Singh, PhD

Dr. Vijendra Singh is a leader in the field of neurobiology and immunology research with more than 100 scientific publications. A researcher at Utah State University, he has focused on central nervous system disorders throughout his career. He is an authority on autoimmunity in autism and related brain disorders.

This chapter contains technical material.

The World Health Organization (WHO) recently announced that brain disorders and mental illnesses are the number one health problems facing people today. No one knows all the causes for these problems, and the financial burden to cope with them surpasses all other conditions including heart disease and cancer. One explanation might be an autoimmune response driven by environmental factors, says Dr. Singh. He explained for ACN:

SEVERAL YEARS AGO, I COMPLETED A REVIEW ARTICLE that may be of some interest: "Immunotherapy for Brain Diseases and Mental Illnesses" (*Progress in Drug Research* 1997; 48:129-46:Monograph Series). I am convinced that the immune system is important, not just for the nervous system, but for addressing any disease in the body. To give an example, until recently we did not know that cardiac diseases involved an immune response. Now there is good evidence that supports the role of an inflammatory response in heart disease, which may be triggered by a pathogen, such as a virus or bacterium. And inflammation is nothing but an abnormal immune response. I'm suggesting that the immune system plays a central role in the normal health of our body, and the nervous system is hugely affected by the immune response. I have a list of nervous system diseases where either brief reports or extensive research connects them to immune pathogenesis and treatment. Included in the list are conditions such as autism, obsessive-compulsive disorder (OCD), multiple sclerosis, Alzheimer's disease, schizophrenia, and major depression.

About 15 years ago, I tried to communicate my theory of the role of the immune system in Alzheimer's disease. People listened but were not convinced; their frequent response was "What? Tied to the immune system? No way!" But as research has progressed, it has become quite clear that immune factors contribute to Alzheimer's disease—this has resulted both from my own research as well as the research of others. At recent conferences I've attended I have been pleased to find that peers now endorse and recognize the pioneering effort involved in my research. Ten to twelve years after my original studies, others are finding the same autoimmune associations, for example, the

---

Major Breakthrough for TS Research

Editor: The role played by the immune system in Tourette syndrome, tic disorders, and OCD should gain research momentum because of recent publication of a landmark study by James F. Leckman, MD, and colleagues at the Child Study Center of Yale University. They found elevated levels of inflammatory cytokines (IL-12 and TNF-alpha) in TS patients at baseline, and these levels were further elevated after symptom increases. This is an excellent sign of immune activity in TS patients who are known to harbor antibodies to brain region basal ganglia. This study provides a new clue connecting immune activation to autoimmunity. Interestingly, similar immune changes have been found in autism, but Dr. Singh suspects that there would be important differences between these disorders. He considers Dr. Leckman's finding a major breakthrough for research and treatment in TS. (See Leckman JF, Katsovich L, Kawikova I, et al: Increased serum levels of interleukin-12 and tumor necrosis factor-alpha in Tourette's syndrome. *Psychiatry* 2005;57:667-73.)

---

finding of autoantibodies to beta-amyloid protein-(1-40), which is a protein believed to be pathogenetically linked to Alzheimer's disease.[2]

As our knowledge increases, we begin to understand more about the nervous system, and in that context, the immune system has taken on a central role.[1-3] In addition to being linked to autism and Alzheimer's disease, immune factors such as autoimmunity have also been linked to Tourette's syndrome, tic disorder, and OCD.[5] *Streptococcus* infections are being studied in relation to OCD and certain cases of Tourette syndrome, although a great deal remains to be investigated. Our own current research focuses on an autism and autoimmunity connection. I think research into autoimmunity might show some interesting similarities between autism, OCD and Tourette's syndrome. For example, patients with these disorders have antibodies to the basal ganglia region of the brain,[4, 5] and they also harbor elevated levels of interleukin-12,[6, 7] a protein in immune cells that plays a key role in setting up autoimmune diseases.

When questioned on how to identify the nature of immune problems, Dr. Singh suggested:

The immunologic evaluation of patients includes a battery of tests or an immune panel. The correct tests should be requested and, just as important, results must be properly interpreted. The interpretation of results of immune tests is not an easy task; it requires extensive knowledge and experience in clinical immunology and immunodiagnostics. Some of the tests to request are: *serum immunoglobulin* and *immunoglobulin subclasses,* blood lymphocyte count, and different lymphocytes, such as *T- or B-lymphocytes, NK cells,* etc. Currently, there are also some research-oriented tools and special cytokines that have been identified as mediators of the immune process, and they should be examined as well. Two of these cytokines are *interferon-gamma* and *interleukin-12,* the latter of which has especially been regarded by many immunologists as the initiator in the early stages of the autoimmune mechanism; an enforcer, if you like, of early events that cause autoimmunity. According to our extensive laboratory research, autoimmunity in autism may be triggered by a virus infection (eg, an asymptomatic measles infection).[3, 8, 9]

In Tourette syndrome and OCD, a microbial infection, such as a *Streptococcus* infection, might drive autoimmunity, but very little is known in this regard at the moment. Also, autoantibodies need to be identified, and they should be organ-specific. For example, when there has been nervous system involvement, we should then find brain autoantibodies. Furthermore, specificity might be based on which particular part of the brain is involved. The brain is made up of many cells, mainly neurons and glia. This raises another question. Is it the neurons or is it the glial cells that are involved? Is it the myelin-producing cells that are affected? Those questions can be addressed by an analysis of the brain autoantibodies. The most important question then is: What triggers that misguided autoimmune response? Is it an environmental factor, such as a virus, bacterium, or pollutant? That needs to be determined, and we can accomplish finding the answer through blood tests for some of the agents.

Summary Remarks

Concluded from immunology research worldwide, autoimmunity appears to be the core of the problem in many patients with autism, OCD, tic disorders or Tourette syndrome. The existence of immune problems and patient responsiveness to treatment with immune therapy strengthens the concept of a pathogenic role for autoimmunity in brain disorders and mental illnesses. This concept certainly appears to be the case for autism, a finding which led me, in 2000, to designate an autoimmune subset as the "Autoimmune Autistic Disorder." Likewise, other neurologic disorders, such as OCD, Tourette syndrome or tic disorders, are also showing signs of involvement with autoimmunity. Many patients afflicted with these disorders show positive outcomes to treatment with immune modulation therapy.[13, 14] As more and more experimental research continues to pile up evidence in favor of this mechanism, autoimmunity research will gain more popularity among researchers and physicians in the field. Hopefully, such results will have a global effect and change the lives of millions of people suffering from these brain disorders and mental illnesses. *(See the Appendix for Dr. Singh's references.)*

Testing for Autoimmunity in Autism and Neurologic Disorders
Vijendra K. Singh, PhD

Dr. Singh recommends autoimmunity testing in neurological disorders. Although his focus has been on autism, he suggests that autoimmunity also should be tested in patients with other neurologic disorders, including OCD, Tourette syndrome, and tic disorders:

Recent advances have clearly shown that autoimmunity plays a significant role in the pathogenesis of neurologic disorders, including autism, tic disorders and Tourette syndrome. Because the brain is the affected organ, the autoimmune response will be directed to the brain. Autoimmunity is commonly manifested by certain autoimmune factors that we have identified in children with autism and other related neurologic disorders. These factors are important for identifying a brain-specific autoimmune response. Using blood test results, we can determine whether a patient shows autoimmunity to the brain, whether he or she is a candidate for experimental immune therapy, and whether the response to therapy is effective. Thus, this type of immune evaluation is important in helping patients with neurologic disorders.

The specific tests are listed here:

Brain autoantibody profile: This test detects antibodies to two brain proteins, namely the *myelin basic protein* and *neuron-axon filament proteins*. We have found that the incidence of myelin basic protein autoantibody in the autistic population is markedly higher than that of the normal population; hence, it serves as a primary marker of the autoimmune reaction in autism. In contrast, the incidence of neuron-axon filament proteins antibody in autistic patients is only marginally higher than that of normal controls, making it a secondary marker of choice. It is, however, recommended that the two immune markers be tested simultaneously.[3] Furthermore, patients with autism, OCD, tic disorders and Tourette syndrome also should be tested for autoantibodies to caudate nucleus (anti-Cn) or anti-basal ganglia antibodies.[4, 5]

Virus serology profile: This test measures level of antibodies to viruses such as measles, mumps, rubella, or HHV-6. We have shown that the level of measles antibody is elevated in many autistic children, which could be a sign of a present infection, past infection, or immune reaction to the measles, mumps and rubella vaccine.[3, 9] In case of OCD, tic disorders and Tourette syndrome, the bacterial serology for Streptococcus and bacterial culture is also recommended.

Vaccine serology profile: This test detects antibodies to vaccines such as measles, mumps, and rubella, or diptheria, pertussis, and tetanus. We showed that a significant number of autistic children, but not the control (normal) children, harbor a unique type of measles antibody to measles, mumps, and rubella vaccine. This antibody may represent an abnormal or inappropriate immune reaction to this vaccine and should be tested in relation to autoimmunity in autism or other neurologic disorders.[3, 8]

Cytokine profile: Two cytokines, namely interleukin-12 and interferon gamma play a significant role in causing autoimmune diseases. We have found that these two cytokines are selectively elevated in autistic children, suggesting their role in autoimmunity in autism.[7] Interleukin-12 has also been found to be elevated in patients with Tourette syndrome.[6] Thus, these cytokines should be measured as a sign of altered cellular autoimmunity in patients with autism or other neurologic disorders.

Serotonin and serotonin-receptor antibody profile: This test measures serum or plasma levels of serotonin and antibodies to brain serotonin receptors. We have found that the patients with autism and other neurologic disorders have an abnormal level of serotonin,[11] the level of which should be tested before administering the treatment with selective serotonin reuptake inhibitors (SSRI antidepressants). We have also found antibodies to brain serotonin receptors in patients with autism and OCD.[12] Thus, these should be tested in patients with neurologic problems.

Mercury-induced autoimmune markers: This test assays for autoimmunity to exposure with heavy metals, such as mercury. These markers include antinucleolar antibodies, antilaminin antibodies and antimetallothionein antibodies. (We have found that only a small number of autistic children are positive for these antibodies, but the level of these antibodies did not differ significantly from levels in control healthy children.[10]) Heavy metals can sometimes also trigger autoimmune phenomenon, and, therefore, these markers should be tested in patients with autism, OCD, tic disorders or Tourette syndrome. *(References in Appendix.)*

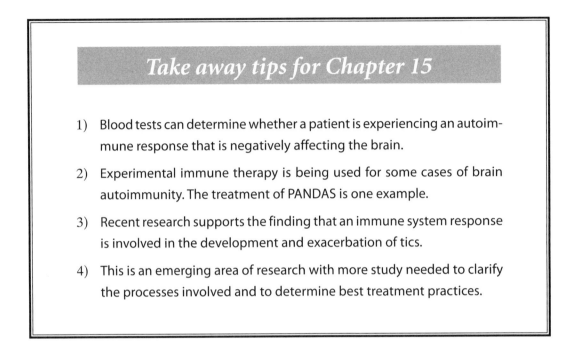

Take away tips for Chapter 15

1) Blood tests can determine whether a patient is experiencing an autoimmune response that is negatively affecting the brain.

2) Experimental immune therapy is being used for some cases of brain autoimmunity. The treatment of PANDAS is one example.

3) Recent research supports the finding that an immune system response is involved in the development and exacerbation of tics.

4) This is an emerging area of research with more study needed to clarify the processes involved and to determine best treatment practices.

Notes:

_____

_____

_____

_____

_____

_____

_____

SECTION FIVE

Diet and Nutrition

CHAPTER

16

The Role of Diet in Tic Disorders

FOR MORE THAN TWENTY YEARS, PARENTS AND CLINICIANS have reported that dietary changes can reduce tics—often dramatically. This is the first book to present this important connection in a comprehensive manner.

It is not unusual for doctors to discourage families from pursuing diet management, and they may even suggest that you would be wasting your time. We can assume that because there is little published information specific to diet and tic disorders, doctors are not aware of this relationship. Foods can affect neurotransmitter function in the brain, as shown in numerous studies, and evidence gathered by ACN indicates that food affects tics. Considering that conventional medicine has so little to offer in the way of helpful treatment for tics, families should be applauded for their efforts to find natural interventions—not dissuaded from exploring dietary changes.

Many of you may already suspect foods as a trigger for tics. In this chapter, we will show you how to determine which specific foods are creating a problem. We'll also discuss the types of foods that support and nourish the nervous system.

In comparison with other movement disorders and conditions that often co-exist with tics (eg, migraine headache, attention deficit hyperactivity disorder [ADHD]), there has been very little attention from the scientific community concerning the effect of nutrition on these disorders. The lists that follow highlight this point; while many of the conditions have significant numbers of studies, tics and Tourette syndrome (TS) have few. *Source: National Library of Medicine, March 2005; computer search for the association of diet and vitamins with the disorders listed:*

Diet	Number of Studies
Depression	1,740
Epilepsy	698
Multiple sclerosis	159
Migraine	143
Parkinson's disease	126
ADHD	90
Tardive dyskinesia *(see note)*	20
Tics	6
Tourette syndrome	5

Vitamins	Number of Studies
Epilepsy	1,446
Depression	1,101
Parkinson's disease	282
Multiple sclerosis	235
Tardive dyskinesia *(see note)*	86
Migraine	80
ADHD	35
Tics	5
Tourette syndrome	4

Note: Tardive dyskinesia is a serious movement disorder that can develop from the use of select drugs prescribed to treat tics.

Finding and coping with food sensitivities

A dietary approach to eliminating or decreasing tics falls into two areas: One is avoiding foods that make symptoms worse, and the other is including nutrient-rich foods your body and brain need to function properly. We will address both of these areas, with the understanding that specific nutritional needs for people with tics or TS have not yet been formally identified.

We should never underestimate the effect food can have on all body systems. Consider this: A slice of aged cheese can trigger an excruciating migraine headache; foods colored with Yellow Dye #5 have sent people with asthma rushing to the hospital emergency department; and a tiny amount of the common peanut can kill a highly allergic person within minutes. It should not be surprising that foods and the chemical additives in foods can also trigger tics.

By eating the proper foods, you can help correct nutritional imbalances and reduce sensitivities. However, you need to first learn which diet is right for you. Sometimes an improvement in tic symptoms results from making just a few changes, such as eliminating caffeine and artificial additives while adding essential fatty acids and magnesium. Another example would be adding high-protein foods and reducing sugars while taking B-vitamins and digestive enzymes. Yet, in many cases, a comprehensive approach is needed to identify specific dietary and nutritional supplement needs.

Common problem foods

Foods most commonly reported as causing negative neurologic reactions, based on reports by several allergists, were listed in an article in the *Annals of Allergy* by Dr. M. B. Campbell. We have summarized the list in order, starting with the most frequently reported food. Many additional foods could also be involved.

Foods commonly reported to cause a neurologic reaction:

1) Milk
2) Wheat
3) Egg
4) Corn
5) Chocolate
6) Beef
7) Potato
8) Coffee
9) Citrus
10) Beans
11) Also: select spices, shellfish, fish, tomato, pork, and lettuce

Other foods widely reported to cause a variety of symptoms in susceptible people include peanuts (a legume), nuts (ie, cashews, walnuts), and soy. Artificial flavors, food colorings, preservatives, monosodium glutamate (MSG), and aspartame are also often problematic.

This does not mean that one or more of these foods are aggravating symptoms for everyone with tics, nor that they are the only ones that may be bothersome. You will have to experiment or pursue evaluations to learn more about your own sensitivities.

John H. Boyles, MD, on food allergy

Dr. John Boyles, past president of the Pan American Allergy Society and an environmental physician in practice in Centerville, Ohio, gave ACN the following explanation about the causes of food allergies and why they can be difficult to detect.

Dr. Boyles:

There are two types of food allergy: fixed and cyclic. Fixed food allergies account for 5% of allergies and are usually *IgE mediated.* (IgE is a type of antibody in the blood.) These sensitivities are obvious to the patient because ingestion of the food produces extreme reactions. A common example is peanut allergy.

In contrast, cyclic food allergy develops over a variable period and is usually a reaction to foods that are eaten repeatedly and/or to foods for which some people are not well adapted, such as dairy and grains. Although a food may enter and exit the body within 24 to 36 hours (the gastrointestinal passage time) associated allergic reactions can persist up to four to five days.

If one is allergic to a food that is eaten only once or twice a month, the allergy reaction is fairly obvious, enabling the patient to make a self-diagnosis. However, when an allergy develops to a food that is eaten every day, because that food is always present in the body, the person has no idea what is causing the problem. These idiopathic reactions (of unknown origin), combined with other sensitivities, such as allergy to substances that are inhaled and chemical sensitivity, produce a confusing picture that the patient cannot easily understand. A second mechanism makes self-diagnosis even more confusing. The initial allergy response can stimulate the brain, causing a pleasant feeling at first which is later followed by a letdown. This pleasant feeling is why people tend to eat more of the foods to which they are allergic. To achieve a sense of mental alertness, the person tends to repeatedly eat the allergic foods, while other organ systems slowly deteriorate. In essence, the person becomes addicted to the very foods that are causing problems.

> It is important to remember that food allergy is dynamic. The more frequently a food is eaten, the more likely it is that the allergy or sensitivity will worsen.

It is important to remember that food allergy is dynamic. The more frequently a food is eaten, the more likely it is that the allergy or sensitivity will worsen. Conversely, the longer the food is eliminated from the diet, the more likely the individual will become tolerant of the food, eventually allowing the food to be included in the diet on a rotation basis.

Elimination diets can help pinpoint problems

As Dr. Boyles explained, it can be difficult to identify all the foods that can trigger reactions in the body. The *elimination diet* is considered the most reliable method for determining troublesome foods because of its ability to expose reactions to specific foods. However, pursuing the diet requires an organized effort on the part of the patient and the patient's family

In the elimination diet, select foods are not eaten in any form for several days. For example, a diet that eliminates corn and milk avoids whole corn, corn syrup, cornmeal, cornstarch, corn flour, popcorn—and any processed products containing these. Milk and milk products in all forms would also not be eaten. The eliminated foods are reintroduced, one by one, on separate days to see whether they cause symptoms. In this case, to reintroduce corn, a significant amount of corn and corn products would be eaten on one day. A few days later, milk, cheese, and other milk products are eaten. Reintroducing the eliminated food is called a *challenge*. A reaction should occur during or soon after the challenge if the dieter is sensitive to that food. *Caution: If prone to significant food reactions, arrange to conduct a challenge in the presence of a nurse or physician who can treat an allergic response.* If you already know of particular foods that are bothersome, do not test a reaction to them and do not eat them during the diet.

Doris J. Rapp, MD, suggests in her new book, *Our Toxic World,* that one way to decide which foods to eliminate is to make a list of several favorite foods and two favorite beverages as a starting point. You can also take the list provided on page 175 and investigate these foods as possible triggers.

Self-education and consultation with a professional can help in determining which type of diet is most appropriate for you. Books on the subject include lists of food families, synonyms of food ingredients to help with label-reading (such as *lactose,* which is milk sugar), and other relevant details. *Food Allergies and Food Intolerance: The Complete Guide to Their Identification and Treatment* by Jonathan Brostoff, MD, is an excellent and thorough text for this purpose.

Clinical methods of food allergy testing and treatment

Besides trying a food elimination diet, another way to uncover the food substances to which one is allergic is to do blood tests, skin tests, and other types of evaluations. These tests include the r*adio allergosorbent test* (RAST) blood test, the *enzyme-linked immunosorbent assay* (ELISA) blood test (for immediate and/or delayed reactions), the *skin prick test*, the *intradermal skin test*, and *enzyme potentiated desensitization* (also known as *low-dose immunotherapy*). See also energy medicine, pages 248–249.

The type of allergy treatment that appears to be most successful for tics, based on reports to ACN, is *optimal dose/neutralization immunotherapy*. This approach is used by many allergists belonging to the American Academy of Environmental Medicine (www.aaem.com). This method of immunotherapy, based on intradermal skin testing, allows for symptom relief without using a "build-up" of dosage common in conventional allergy therapy; many people with sensitivities to foods and chemicals cannot tolerate build-up. The neutralization treatment serves to help relieve current symptoms while also reducing the likelihood of future reactions. The injections are safe and can usually be administered at home by injection; sublingual drops are sometimes used. Special training of allergy technicians is required for appropriate diagnosis and treatment. (Inhalant allergy can also be treated in this manner.)

Although ACN knows other allergy management to be useful for some people, there is not yet sufficient data to report on them.

Milk- and wheat-free diets

The top two foods reported to cause neurologic reactions are milk and wheat. Let's examine the concept of milk- and wheat-free diets, as well as gluten sensitivity, an offshoot of wheat allergy.

Milk allergy: The immune system can respond negatively to milk, creating an allergic reaction, and sensitivity to the carbohydrates in milk can result in lactose intolerance. Another type of negative response, a reaction to the specific milk protein, *casein*, is not as well-known and is more difficult to detect. When casein is improperly digested, it breaks down into peptides that get into the bloodstream and cross into the brain, where they can cause neurologic problems. This biochemical reaction has been linked to autism, and this is the reason that a milk-free diet has helped many of these youngsters. Families that avoid dairy can usually substitute rice, soy (in moderation), or nut milks unless sensitivities to these foods exist as well.

Wheat and gluten allergy: A wheat allergy involves adverse reactions to protein substances in wheat. Avoiding wheat often solves the problem. However, when the problem is an intolerance to the gluten in wheat, that person may need to avoid other grains (oats, barley, rye, and triticale) that also contain gluten. A blood test for gluten sensitivity can often determine whether gluten is a problem. Although some experts suggest oats are gluten-free and may be tolerated, others have concern that oats may be cross-contaminated with other gluten-containing grains and therefore should be avoided by the highly sensitive. Spelt, promoted as a "wheat alternative," also contains gluten. Flours that do not contain gluten are made from rice, corn (cornmeal), millet, potato, tapioca, quinoa, buckwheat, amaranth, teff, nuts, sorghum, and beans, among others.

> William H. Philpott, MD, author of *Brain Allergy*, informed ACN through personal correspondence that in his clinical practice he has found that a gluten-free diet is often helpful for reducing tics.

William H. Philpott, MD, author of *Brain Allergy*, informed ACN through personal correspondence that in his clinical practice he has found that a gluten-free diet is often helpful for reducing tics. This observation has been reinforced by sporadic reports to ACN received from patients and families.

Cutting out chemical additives in foods: The Feingold Program

Benjamin F. Feingold, MD (1900-1982), a pediatrician and allergist, encouraged removing synthetic food dyes and flavorings from the diet because he found they could cause behavioral and learning problems. He later added preservatives (ie, BHA, BHT,

Celiac Disease and Tics

We were interested in research published in 2004 on *Celiac disease* that mentions tics. It was completed in Israel by Nattie Zelnik, MD, and colleagues. Celiac disease, an autoimmune condition involving a serious gluten allergy, is treated by following a strict gluten-free diet. This condition was once considered rare in North America but is now more common, as is true of some other modern autoimmune conditions.

Dr. Zelnik's team studied Celiac disease in more than 100 children, adolescents, and young adults to learn how common it is for them to also have neurologic conditions, such as headache, learning disorders, ADHD, and tic disorders. Study results show that patients with Celiac disease are significantly more prone to develop neurologic disorders than those without the condition (the control group). These disorders include decreased muscle tone, developmental delay, learning disorders and ADHD, headache, and a disorder of the nervous system affecting balance and coordination.

Interestingly, the only condition that was studied for which there were *fewer* symptoms among those with Celiac disease compared with the control group was tics. We wondered—could it be that the group with Celiac disease was following a gluten-free diet and this intervention helped prevent the development of tics? We contacted Dr. Zelnik for his opinion on this idea, and he replied (March 2005):

"As you mentioned in your correspondence, we did not find a higher prevalence of tics among patients with Celiac disease in comparison with the control group. This was a bit of a surprise to us, but this is what we found. Your suggestion that perhaps the gluten-free diet prevented the occurrence of tics is possible. Nevertheless I would be cautious in drawing such a conclusion, as even among patients who were diagnosed late (and lived for years without restriction of gluten), we were unable to show a higher prevalence of tics."

Additional research on this topic would be valuable. We request readers dealing with a tic disorder who have had testing completed for gluten sensitivity, or who have experimented with a gluten-free diet, to please contact ACN, PO Box 210848, Royal Palm Beach, FL 33421-0848. Input from medical practitioners is also appreciated. All contacts are confidential.

TBHQ) to the list of offenders. Dr. Feingold also discovered that *salicylate*, a natural occurring substance in some foods, affected some, though fewer in number. Salicylate is chemically related to aspirin, which is a derivative of salicylic acid. Some people are reportedly only troubled by one or two foods that contain salicylate, while others are sensitive to all of them. Foods containing salicylate include raisins, grapes, berries, cucumbers and peppers, among a number of other fruits and vegetables, and other select foods.

Dr. Feingold's efforts evolved into the Feingold Association of the United States (FAUS), a nonprofit organization that promotes his message. According to FAUS, most food colors have not been studied for their effect on the brain and nervous system, and only new additives are now being studied for neurotoxicity.

Jane Hersey, director of FAUS, advised ACN: "Muscles and nerves appear to be especially sensitive to the effects of certain synthetic food additives—particularly dyes, artificial flavors, the synthetic sweetener aspartame (NutraSweet), monosodium glutamate (MSG), and some preservatives. Our organization has received many reports from members who observe a connection between additives and tics. When the additives are removed from the diet, a marked improvement in tic symptoms is seen. I would encourage anyone dealing with tics to explore the possible role of synthetic additives in the diet."

> "Muscles and nerves appear to be especially sensitive to the effects of certain synthetic food additives—particularly dyes, artificial flavors, the synthetic sweetener aspartame (NutraSweet), monosodium glutamate (MSG), and some preservatives."
>
> —Jane Hersey

It's a misconception among the medical community that only a small percentage of sensitive people may be bothered by these additives. Studies suggest otherwise. The results of research in 2004 conducted by Dr. Belinda J. Bateman and colleagues showed that even "normal" children can become hyperactive when fed artificial food colorings and preservatives. On the basis of these findings, the researchers recommend that all chemical additives be removed from foods.

The food industry is starting to respond to a growing public demand by offering more all-natural, additive-free food products. The Feingold Association of the United States (*www.feingold.org*) offers their members comprehensive, updated food lists of additive-free foods and drinks. The lists save you the trouble of examining every label and provide information about hidden food ingredients that you might not be aware of unless you contacted the manufacturers.

The Food Intolerance Network of Australia provides extensive advice on additive free-diets (available at: *www.fedupwithfoodadditives.info*). This organization focuses on information on a wide range of potentially problematic substances including salycilates and amines (naturally occurring chemicals in foods).

The Hyperactive Children's Support Group in England does an excellent job of sharing information on the Feingold diet and other nutrition-related issues. They also work with schools in the UK, educating teachers on the importance of food as it relates to behavior and academics. Sally Bunday, director, has told ACN that the organization receives reports on the role of diet in regard to tics. The Hyperactive Children's Support Group (*www.hacsg.org.uk*) recommends an additive-free diet with nutrient-rich foods for those with TS and other tic disorders.

A digestive enzyme, *phenol sulfotransferase* (known as PST), can be overloaded by certain petroleum-based additives, interfering with the normal digestive process. This connection has been documented for autism, and targeted enzyme supplementation is increasing in popularity as part of a multidisciplinary approach to autism. (See *www. enzymestuff.com*.)

Sweets and tics

Parents often report to ACN that tic symptoms worsen when their children eat sweets. For this reason, along with eliminating additives as an important step in adjusting the diet, reducing the amount of cane sugar and other sweeteners, such as corn syrup, maple syrup, fructose, and honey, is recommended. Those who react negatively to sweets should also minimize their intake of fruit juices and dried fruits.

Controversy over the role sugar plays in health and behavior has been confusing to the public. One source of the conflict is rooted in the lack of distinction made between the terms *sweets* and *sugar*. Although parents report that sugar makes behavior worse, some studies that have received major media attention indicate that "sugar" does not have any negative affect. Joseph B. Miller, MD, author of *Relief at Last! Neutralization for Food Allergy and Other Illnesses*, offered ACN this explanation: "Typically, children do not eat plain granulated sugar by the teaspoon, so the response to sugar itself is not likely to be identified. Rather, they eat 'sweets' that are usually produced in food factories, such as candy bars, jelly beans, chewy fruit candies, hard candies, fruit-filled pastries, cinnamon rolls, doughnuts, ice cream, sherbet, jellies and preserves, pancake syrups, sweetened cereals, etc. Researchers are generally studying 'sugar' or sucrose—a single ingredient isolated from dyes, additives, other sweeteners, and chocolate or other ingredients. Parents are reporting that sugar increases tics or hyperactivity, but often they mean sweets, not granulated sugar per se."

Sherry A. Rogers, MD, an environmental physician and author of several books on the subjects of chemical sensitivity and allergy, emphasizes that problems with *glucose control* in the body, particularly low blood sugar (hypoglycemia), should be considered as a possible underlying cause of tics. Glucose is a simple sugar made from carbohydrates in food. Dr. Rogers has seen a connection between tics and glucose dysregulation in her clinical practice and suggests that a glucose tolerance test can help rule out this possibility. Glucose tolerance tests are routine evaluations and can be arranged through a pediatrician, general practitioner, or medical specialist.

Some cases of people having obsessive thoughts, which those with TS often experience, have also been linked to the inability of the body to properly handle glucose. An article in the *British Journal of Clinical Psychology* in 1983 highlighted a chronic case of obsessive or intrusive thoughts that had not responded to years of psychologic and drug therapy. The authors found that the obsessions were not psychologic in nature but rather "a brain dysfunction secondary to nutritional factors." This patient made a dramatic and lasting recovery when a high-protein breakfast was added to the diet. A high-protein diet helps to balance the body's blood sugar levels. Other studies have explored glucose metabolism in obsessive-compulsive disorder and their results support consideration of this glucose connection for at least a subgroup of people.

> Some cases of people having obsessive thoughts, which those with TS often experience, have been linked to the inability of the body to properly handle glucose.

Sugar substitutes

It may be tempting to replace sugars with the popular artificial sweetener, aspartame (sold under trade names such as Nutrasweet, Spoonful, and Equal). Beware, however.

H. J. Roberts, MD, author of the recent *Defense Against Alzheimer's Disease*, has crusaded about the dangers of aspartame since the 1980s. Dr. Roberts' research database suggests that potential reactions to aspartame are grossly underestimated in both severity and scope in conventional literature. He notes that most physicians often encounter reactions to aspartame but, unaware of the underlying problem, do not inquire about aspartame use. According to Dr. Roberts, the negative effects of aspartame potentially link to such problems as aggravation of diabetes mellitus, hypoglycemia, convulsions, headache, depression, other psychiatric states, hyperthyroidism, hypertension, arthritis, multiple sclerosis, Alzheimer's disease, and lupus erythematosus, among others.

It should be pointed out that most research studies to date suggest that aspartame is safe in moderate amounts. Dr. Roberts warns, however, that toxic effects to the brain can occur when products with aspartame have been in prolonged storage or are exposed to high temperatures (above 86° F.). He asserts that when research is done on aspartame, it is not done using heated or "old" aspartame; therefore, these problems are not encountered and, thus, not published.

> Research shows that aspartame consumption can cause neurologic problems; in high doses, it can lower the threshold for seizure activity. If aspartame can lower the threshold for seizures, it is reasonable to suspect that it can also lower the threshold for tics.

According to feedback received by ACN, some people identify aspartame—now an ingredient in 5,000 products—as a trigger for their tics. And research shows that aspartame consumption can cause neurologic problems; in high doses, it can lower the threshold for seizure activity. If aspartame can lower the threshold for seizures, it is reasonable to suspect that it can also lower the threshold for tics. We therefore recommend that products with aspartame be avoided. Instead, consider using the herbal extract, stevia. A natural sugar substitute, stevia is 300 times sweeter than sugar without the high calories, and it has some beneficial properties. Stevia is sold as a food, not as a sweetener, and is found in most natural grocery stores. Long-term human studies support its use in moderate amounts as a sugar substitute.

Other sugar substitutes now on the market, such as sorbitol and mannitol, are made by adding hydrogen atoms to sugar. Although many people reportedly tolerate these substitutes, they sometimes cause gas, bloating, and diarrhea, even when consumed in relatively small amounts. Xylitol, a naturally occurring substance, is used in chewing gum and has been shown to reduce the development of dental caries. It is sold in bulk as XyloSweet and can be used in a manner similar to sugar. Xylitol products do not affect blood sugar levels as rapidly as regular sugar and have fewer calories per teaspoon than sugar. Saccharin (Sweet'N Low), an old standby, has been reported to be associated with increased cancer risk since the late 1970s, but these reports have remained controversial. Sucralose (Splenda) is made when natural sugar is restructured using chlorine atoms. This popular artificial sweetener has not yet been well-tested. Even less is known about a new sweetener, Tagatose (Naturlose), which is made from lactose, a milk sugar.

Yeast overgrowth: *Candida albicans*

All types of regular (not artificial) sweets or sweeteners are reported to increase *Candida albicans*, a natural yeast that is present in everyone's body. When it is kept in check, it is harmless. However, when it grows out of control, the result can be adverse reactions to foods and many other health problems.

Friendly intestinal bacteria such as *Bifidobacteria bifidum* and *Lactobaccillus acidophilus* typically provide a balance to keep *C albicans* and other yeasts in check. Besides improper diet and sweets, antibiotics, birth control pills, nutritional deficiencies, corticosteroids, and immune deficiencies can allow *C albicans* to increase out of control, resulting in an imbalance in intestinal flora. One consequence of this overgrowth is leaky gut syndrome, in which the lining of the intestinal tract is damaged, allowing food-related substances to enter the bloodstream and create numerous health problems. *C albicans* overgrowth can play a significant role in ADHD, OCD, depression, tic disorders, and autism. Please see Chapter 18 on *C albicans* that includes interviews with William G. Crook, MD, and William Shaw, PhD, for a more technical discussion of this topic; advice on what you can do to restore the proper intestinal balance is included.

The macrobiotic diet

Michio Kushi and Alex Jack recommend a *macrobiotic diet* for those with TS in their book, *The Macrobiotic Path to Total Health*. In macrobiotics, emphasis is placed on whole grains, select vegetables in season, protein foods (beans, soy products, or fish to account for about 10% of the diet), a small amount of sea vegetables (kombu, nori, and other seaweeds), soups, fruits, nuts, seeds, and beverages. Dairy products are excluded, as are sugars and sweets, alcohol, coffee, and meats. A successful case report on TS and the macrobiotic diet is provided by the authors. The underlying theory purported about this individual's success is that the patient was formally eating too much meat, especially chicken, as well as an excess of spices, sugar, and stimulants. ACN has received a small number of positive reports from adults who have said the macrobiotic diet was helpful; no research has yet been completed.

As with other restricted food plans, pregnant or nursing mothers and young children need to be assured of adequate nutrition. Having said that, the macrobiotic diet's emphasis on eating nutritious, natural foods and avoiding sugars and stimulants is compatible with other helpful dietary approaches reported to ACN.

The rotation diet

Many of us eat the same foods repeatedly. For example, meals containing wheat, dairy, corn, and tomatoes are often eaten every day in one form or another. One method to help a person avoid this repetitive ingestion of foods is to follow a *rotation diet*. With the rotation diet, foods that are the most troublesome are not allowed, and other foods are rotated throughout the week, never having a particular food or other foods from its group more often than every four days. For example, if you eat soy on Monday, you would not eat anything containing soy again until Friday.

Research supports the use of the rotation diet as a treatment for multiple food sensitivities when gastrointestinal issues are involved. When foods are causing symptoms, a rotation diet, also known as a rotary diversified elimination diet, can help reduce symptoms and allow more foods to be integrated into the diet. It also allows for easier identification of troublesome foods and helps prevent the development of new sensitivities.

Books on rotation diets offer lists of food families so you can plan what foods can be eaten each day. This is a challenging diet and requires self-education and ongoing support to maintain it. People sometimes ask, "Who would want to go to all the trouble of going on this diet?" The answer is: someone who is unable to find relief from food sensitivities through other methods.

Pesticides and the Nervous System
Joseph T. Rogers, DO

Joseph T. Rogers, DO, a cardiologist and environmental physician at Downriver Cardiology in Trenton, Michigan, explained the impact of two common types of pesticides:

Organophosphates and *carbamates,* can have acute effects on the *cholinergic enzyme system*. Under normal conditions, an impulse passes from nerve to nerve with the aid of a chemical transmitter called *acetylcholine*. This transmitting chemical is necessary to the normal functioning of the body. If the acetylcholine is not destroyed as soon as a nerve impulse has passed, impulses continue to flash across the bridge from nerve to nerve as the acetylcholine exerts its effects in an evermore intensifying manner. Potentially, the movements of the whole body can become uncoordinated; tremors, muscle spasms, convulsions, and even death can result. Normally a protective enzyme called *cholinesterase* is at hand to destroy the transmitting chemical once it is no longer needed. By this means, a precise balance is struck and the body never builds up a dangerous amount of acetylcholine. However, on contact with an organophosphate or carbamate insecticide, the protective enzyme is destroyed; as the quantity of the enzyme is reduced, that of the transmitting chemical builds up.

Scientists from the FDA discovered that for certain *organophosphates*, when two are administered simultaneously, the compound can be up to fifty times as potent as would be predicted on the basis of adding together the toxicities of each of the two. Aldicarb (a carbamate) poisoning from treated foods may include common influenza symptoms, eye-twitching, other muscular twitching, weakness, disorientation, hyperexcitability, and even death. Pesticides and fungicides have been implicated in Parkinson's disease.

Considering the documented relationship between pesticides and central nervous system reactions, it is a reasonable concern that tics could be aggravated by exposure to pesticides, even at low levels. It is recommended that individuals with these conditions eat organic food when feasible. Consumers should be particularly wary of produce from Central and South America where regulation of pesticide use is notoriously lax. Further, it is suggested that personal use of toxic pesticides inside and outside the home be restricted and replaced with more environmentally-sound products.

Pesticides and processed foods

Many agree that modern diets are lacking in the required nutrients and that the so-called "balanced diet" is rarely consumed. Harold E. Buttram, MD, points out: "Today, only the older generation can remember the pattern of sit-down family meals prepared with simple, unprocessed foods. Nutritionists estimate that today's highly processed foods may have less than 20% of the vital nutrients of foods in earlier times. Good nutrition is not necessarily more expensive, but it does require a return to simple, unadulterated foods."

While focusing on eating a variety of nutritious foods, we should also focus on including organic foods in our diet whenever possible. Commonly used pesticides can damage the human nervous system, and some foods have been treated with pesticides at levels that exceed federal guidelines. Authorities now agree that guidelines for pesticide use were never properly determined for children. Such guidelines also do not take into account that when combined, pesticides are exponentially more harmful than when used alone.

The safest fruits and vegetables

Organic foods are ideal; however it is not always possible to "go organic" because items are more readily available in some areas than in others, and they are frequently expensive. Natural food stores often carry organic grains, beans, and other staple foods which may be moderately priced, as well as organic fresh produce, which tends to be more costly. Fortunately, many standard grocery stores now stock organic foods.

The Environmental Working Group released a wallet-sized shopper's guide to the pesticides in conventional produce. The organization maintains that eating according to these guidelines can reduce the number of pesticides ingested by up to 90%. (See next page.)

In October 2003, the Environmental Working Group (*www.ewg.org*), a leading environmental advocacy organization based in Washington, DC, released a wallet-sized shopper's guide to the pesticides in conventional produce. The organization maintains that eating according to these guidelines can reduce the number of pesticides ingested by up to 90%. The guide lists 12 popular fruits and vegetables that are consistently the most and the least contaminated with pesticides.

Highest in pesticides	*Lowest in pesticides*
Apples	Asparagus
Bell peppers	Avocados
Celery	Bananas
Cherries	Broccoli
Grapes (imported)	Cauliflower
Nectarines	Corn (sweet)
Peaches	Kiwi
Pears	Mangos
Potatoes	Onions
Red raspberries	Papaya
Spinach	Pineapples
Strawberries	Sweet peas

What *should* we eat and drink?

It is essential to eat natural, health-promoting foods that help strengthen our immune system, keep blood sugar levels steady, and provide needed nutrients. Eating right is not complicated, but the diets in more developed countries are often so removed from a natural diet that it takes conscious effort to regain a healthy balance. When reading the suggestions that follow, you must take into consideration your food sensitivities, allergies, or other medical problems, if any.

Include healthful oils

The no-fat diet craze, started by weight loss gurus and fueled by concerns of heart disease, left bodies starving for essential fatty acids. To bring such oil into the diet, we should use moderate amounts of flaxseed oil, canola oil, and olive oil. Purchase organic oils when you can, and buy only extra-virgin olive oils. Look for cold-pressed oils, which have not been subjected to damaging heat, and watch expiration dates. Pumpkin seed, walnut, and safflower oils are also good, and peanut oil remains stable at high cooking temperatures.

Avoid cottonseed oil, which is often mixed with other oils and added to many nuts during roasting. Oils often recommended for use as a supplement include unrefined coconut oil (which can also be used in cooking), cod liver oil or fish oil, flaxseed oil, borage oil, and evening primrose oil. See pages 198-200 on essential fatty acids. Avoid all hydrogenated and partially hydrogenated oils, or *trans fats*.

The best antioxidant-rich foods

Antioxidants help repair damage from disease-causing free radicals in the body, and they also can strengthen the immune system. In 2004, the US Department of Agriculture released results of a study of 100 foods, indicating which ones had the highest levels of antioxidants. Blueberries, cranberries, and blackberries ranked highest among the fruits. Beans, artichokes, and Russet potatoes were the top vegetables/legumes. Pecans, walnuts, and hazelnuts ranked highest in the nut category. When considering the items on this list, also check the list on the preceding page to avoid potential pesticide exposure (eg, strawberries) in conventional foods.

The top 20 foods as measured by total antioxidant capacity per serving size.

1. Small red beans
2. Wild blueberries
3. Red kidney beans
4. Pinto beans
5. Cultivated blueberries
6. Cranberries
7. Artichoke hearts (cooked)
8. Blackberries
9. Prunes
10. Raspberries
11. Strawberries
12. Red delicious apples
13. Granny Smith apples
14. Pecans
15. Sweet cherries
16. Black plums
17. Russet potatoes
18. Black beans
19. Plums
20. Gala apples

Protein and carbohydrates

Although no diet is ideal for everyone, we all need protein and carbohydrates. Despite the current no-carbohydrate fad, some carbohydrates are necessary for energy. Don't fall for the hype that you should not eat any carbs. However, do take note of the huge difference between an iced doughnut, a baked potato, and a bowl of lentil soup—all loaded with carbohydrates. Pick carbohydrates with natural fiber and include some in your diet every day. Good carbs include peas, beans, lentils, and other legumes; carrots, cauliflower, peppers, and potatoes; whole grains as cereals and whole grain flours; nuts and seeds, as well as fresh fruits (eaten in moderation). Avoid refined carbohydrates and those with added sweeteners: typical breads, pastas, and cereals that contain no whole grain or fiber, hard and soft candies, honey, doughnuts, sweetened cereals, cakes, and fruit juice, as well as processed sugars, dextrose, fructose, and corn syrup.

> Proteins provide important building blocks for your cells and will also help keep your blood sugar levels under control.

Proteins provide important building blocks for your cells and will also help keep your blood sugar levels under control. Vegetarians focus on foods such as beans, lentils, whole grains, natural soy products, cheese or cheese alternatives, nuts, and seeds. Meat eaters typically include poultry, lean meat, fish (locate a pure source, without mercury), and eggs.

Smart beverages

It is wise to drink plenty of water and avoid or minimize use of caffeinated drinks and sweet fruit juices. Green and black teas and some herbal teas have antioxidant properties, but be aware that green and black teas often contain caffeine. Also, watch out for prepared teas that are touted as natural, yet are loaded with corn syrup or sugars. Consider diluting fruit juices or look for unsweetened bottled waters that are only lightly flavored with fruit.

Water makes up 60% of the body and nearly 70% of the brain. Make it a point to find a pure source of water for drinking and cooking. Ordinary tap water in most areas contains contaminants, and some bottled water is not much better. Investigate your local water source, different brands of bottled water, and home water purification systems. Distilled water is the purest form of water but should be stored in glass bottles, not plastic, because it can leach chemicals from the container. If you drink large quantities of distilled water, you need to take mineral supplements to replace beneficial minerals that have been removed during the distillation process along with the contaminants.

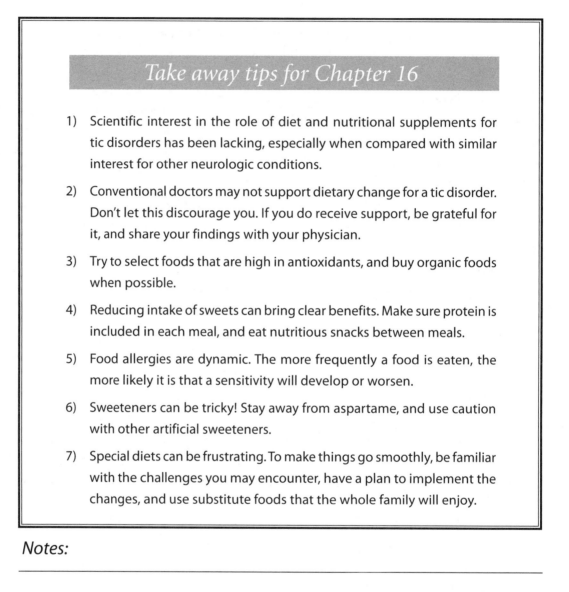

Take away tips for Chapter 16

1) Scientific interest in the role of diet and nutritional supplements for tic disorders has been lacking, especially when compared with similar interest for other neurologic conditions.

2) Conventional doctors may not support dietary change for a tic disorder. Don't let this discourage you. If you do receive support, be grateful for it, and share your findings with your physician.

3) Try to select foods that are high in antioxidants, and buy organic foods when possible.

4) Reducing intake of sweets can bring clear benefits. Make sure protein is included in each meal, and eat nutritious snacks between meals.

5) Food allergies are dynamic. The more frequently a food is eaten, the more likely it is that a sensitivity will develop or worsen.

6) Sweeteners can be tricky! Stay away from aspartame, and use caution with other artificial sweeteners.

7) Special diets can be frustrating. To make things go smoothly, be familiar with the challenges you may encounter, have a plan to implement the changes, and use substitute foods that the whole family will enjoy.

Notes:

_____

_____

_____

_____

17

Nutritional Therapy

MANY TIC DISORDERS RESPOND TO TREATMENT with nutritional supplements. However, the effort is often hit-and-miss because patients and families don't know where to turn for advice. Many hope for a one-size-fits-all answer—a few supplements that can be taken in place of or added to a regimen that includes a prescription drug or drugs. Although nutritional therapy holds great promise, no standardized plan will work for everyone. This chapter highlights both the complexity and the exciting potential of this approach.

Aside from the issue of side effects, conventional medications are convenient because they usually work quickly. Sometimes a trial of just a few days or a few weeks will indicate whether or not a drug is working, and if not, a different one can be tried. Nutritional therapy, on the other hand, does not work that quickly. Yet, when properly followed, it has the benefit of bringing long-lasting results with less concern for side effects. To achieve improvements, a balanced combination of vitamins, minerals, amino acids, essential fatty acids, and other nutrients may be needed.

The role of nutrients in psychiatric disease

In the 1950s, Abram Hoffer, MD, PhD, a noted psychiatrist, in collaboration with

Humphrey Osmond, MD, discovered that some people have nutritional "dependencies," meaning that they require greater levels of one or more nutrients than is typical for other people. They also found they could help correct imbalances in the brains of individuals with schizophrenia by using large doses of specific nutrients, such as vitamin B_3. This was the beginning of "megavitamin" therapy. Nobel Prize winner Linus Pauling (1901–1994) embraced the concept of megavitamin therapy which he renamed "orthomolecular" medicine in the 1960s. He proposed that we can protect our health and treat disease by using varying concentrations of substances that are naturally present in the body. The term *orthomolecular* relates to using the "right molecules in the right concentration."

Nutrients for depression, stress, and immune system strengthening

Patients with tics are often advised to reduce stress, because feeling anxious, nervous, pressured, or embarrassed can aggravate tics. Depression, common among people with tic disorders, can increase stress, making it all the harder to deal with the tics. A weak immune system also leaves a person more vulnerable to stress. Numerous nutritional supplements and herbs can calm the nervous system, relieve depression, and strengthen the immune system.

Numerous nutritional supplements and herbs can calm the nervous system, relieve depression, and strengthen the immune system.

A nutritional therapist considers symptoms, medical history, and laboratory results when determining which supplements at which dosages to recommend. Books are listed in the resource section for more in-depth reading on this topic.

Some of the more commonly used supplements that can help boost the immune system and reduce the stress response follow. This is by no means a complete list and is being provided simply as a basic introduction to some key nutrients. It is strongly recommended that patients or caregivers do not use supplements as treatment without consulting a physician or a nutritional therapist skilled in this area. (See recommendations by Jon B. Pangborn, PhD, on laboratory testing in Chapter 19.)

B complex: These important vitamins include vitamin B_1 (thiamin), B_2 (riboflavin), B_3 (niacin), B_5 (pantothenic acid), B_6 (pyridoxine), B_{12} (cobalamin), biotin, folic acid, choline, and PABA (para-aminobenzoic acid). B_6 can enhance the effects of many other

Quotes by Abram Hoffer, MD, PhD
from an Interview with Sheila J. Rogers

I suggest that for any kind of psychiatric behavior disorder, physicians should follow these guidelines: First, determine whether there is any physical disease. Does the patient have diabetes, hypoglycemia, a brain tumor, etc.? Rule out any physical condition. The next thing to tackle is whether there is a major nutritional problem. Is the person deficient, for example, in B_3, B_6, or zinc? Then consider the family tree for allergy or environmental reactions. A large number of the patients I see are allergic to various foods, particularly wheat, milk, and eggs. I have seen many improve just on a four-day rotation diet. So, you look at food allergies. Then look to see if they are eating nutritionally sound food. One cannot compensate for a poor diet by taking huge quantities of supplements.

✢

I define the *optimum dose* as the quantity that restores health without causing either unpleasant or dangerous side effects. Keep in mind, however, that the optimum dose required to restore health may be too high once the patient has recovered; the new maintenance dose will probably be lower. That dose needs to be determined by trial and error. I describe specifics for optimum doses for each nutrient in some of my books. (See below.)

✢

I used to be puzzled by the fact that some children would respond to nutritional therapy and others would not, though both the children's clinical symptoms seemed to be the same. I then learned about cerebral allergies and found that the nonresponders could attain good results once environmental factors and food allergies were also addressed. In addition to recommending adjustments in the environment, another approach orthomolecular medicine uses to address chemical sensitivity is to provide nutrients that will improve the immune system—especially vitamin C, vitamin E, and selenium. We may also use some of the better antihistamines to reduce allergic reactions.

Books by Abram Hoffer: *Orthomolecular Medicine for Physicians; Smart Nutrients: Prevent and Treat Alzheimer's, Enhance Brain Function*; see resources for details.

vitamins and minerals. B vitamins are often depleted by a stress response and need to be replenished. B_{12} supplementation is associated with reduced anxiety and increased energy; inositol, a well-tolerated form of niacin, has shown promise for treating panic disorders, as well as depression and obsessive-compulsive disorder (OCD). Some people have adverse reactions to B-complex preparations and need to address each vitamin separately as they may not tolerate supplementation of all the B vitamins.

Taurine: This amino acid maintains neurotransmitter function in the brain and is essential for a strong immune system and good vision. Taurine deficiency has been linked to seizures. A B_6 deficiency can cause a deficit in taurine levels. A powerful antioxidant, taurine plays a significant role in the body's use of magnesium.

Glutathione: This protein is crucial for removing toxic metals in the body, such as mercury and cadmium and can be helpful in combating depression. It is administered orally, topically in lotion form, or intravenously. Toxins greatly increase stress at the cellular level. (Zinc, selenium, and vitamin C are commonly used to safely reduce levels of toxins in the body.) Books by David Perlmutter, MD: *Brainrecovery.Com: Powerful Therapy for Challenging Brain Disorders* and *The Better Brain Book* describe the use of glutathione for Parkinson's disease and other movement disorders.

Tryptophan: This essential amino acid is important for the body's production of serotonin and melatonin. According to research by David E. Comings, MD, Tourette syndrome (TS) patients have lower levels of tryptophan in the blood than is typical. Tryptophan was an effective and popular antidepressant and sleep aid until the late 1980s. It was banned by the US Federal Drug Administration because a contaminated batch from Japan caused more than 1,000 people to fall ill. This was a serious but isolated problem. Tryptophan (sold as L-tryptophan) is now available again through prescription or from some small nutritional supplement companies. Seek expert advice on the use of this and other amino acids.

 5-HTP (5-Hydroxytryptophan): Another amino acid, 5-HTP, is often used as an antidepressant and remedy for insomnia. It has proven helpful for migraine headaches, among other conditions and is often recommended in place of tryptophan supplementation because it acts in a similar manner yet is easier to obtain.

SAMe (Adenosyl-L-Methionine): SAMe, a natural substance present throughout the body, has been used extensively as an antidepressant supplement.

St. John's wort (Hypericum Performatum): This herbal remedy is one of the most well-known for treating depression. In recent studies, St John's wort was shown to be beneficial for both mild and moderate depression, and it is also used to reduce anxiety and stress. An overview of studies, however, shows mixed results. As with other supplements that affect neurotransmitter function, you should discuss potential side effects with your practitioner.

Antioxidants: Vitamin A, E, and C are often recommended for improving immune functioning. Vitamin C is the most widely researched of this group and is recognized for its important role in reducing inflammation and promoting healing. Coenzyme Q10 (Co-Q10) is a strong antioxidant and can strengthen immune response, improve adrenal gland functioning, and protect against oxidative stress at the cellular level. Zinc and selenium also have antioxidant properties.

Probiotics: Combined with a multivitamin, probiotics are reported to reduce stress and exhaustion and improve the immune system. While *antibiotics* work against harmful bacteria, *probiotics*—such as the acidophilus found in yogurt—are natural substances that work to promote helpful bacteria. Antibiotics upset the balance of bacterial colonies in the digestive tract because at the same time they are eliminating the toxic bacteria, they are also destroying the bacteria that is beneficial. See Chapter 18 for more information on probiotics and how they can help your health.

Minerals: The brain and nervous system rely on a proper balance of minerals that include manganese, calcium, iron, selenium, zinc, and/or copper, among others. An experienced nutritional practitioner can help determine deficiencies of these minerals as well as minerals in overload that may be causing problems (such as an excess of copper).

Magnesium: This essential mineral relaxes nerve impulses, reduces some headaches, and can ease muscle contractions. Muscle spasms are one of several signs of a magnesium deficiency. Researcher Jon B. Pangborn, PhD, suggests that supplementation with magnesium can help eliminate tics in some people. In addition, Bonnie Grimaldi has proposed a theory that magnesium deficiency may be at the root of many cases of TS.

Magnesium can help promote restful sleep, and it assists in removing the toxic metals lead and cadmium from the body. Studies show that many in the general population are deficient in magnesium.

Zinc: This mineral is necessary for proper immune function, action of neurotransmitters, metabolism of essential fatty acids, and maintaining a healthy digestive tract. William Walsh, PhD, indicates that a low-zinc to high-copper ratio has been found in a subgroup of patients with depression, and this abnormal ratio is common among the autistic population. A nutritionally oriented doctor can help you explore this possibility, and provide therapy designed to balance the ratio.

Digestive enzymes: Supplementing with digestive enzymes is not a new concept. However, new versions are more finely tuned and more specific in their action. Taken with meals, enzymes can help protect against food sensitivity reactions by aiding the digestive process. Houston Neutraceuticals (*www.houstonni.com*) and Kirkman Labs (*www.kirkmanlabs.com*) are developing and marketing a range of new plant-based digestive enzymes, and they offer helpful information.

Omega-3 essential fatty acids and tic disorders

Cells in our bodies are surrounded by a membrane composed of fatty compounds derived from *essential fatty acids* (EFAs). Essential fatty acids are crucial for proper nerve receptor formation and transmission in the brain, as well as the exchange of chemical signals in the retina of the eye. Many nutritionists suggest that the standard Western diet has insufficient amounts of "good" fats, such as EFAs. Natural foods that contain healthful fats are often altered by replacing the perishable fats with harmful trans fats to give products a longer shelf life.

The term "essential fatty acids" is used because the body cannot manufacture these fats; they must come from our diet. Interest in EFAs spiked in the late 1990s when Andrew L. Stoll, MD, reported that therapy with fish oil, which is rich in EFAs, had positive results for some cases of bipolar (manic-depressive) disorder. Its benefit was soon documented for ADHD, and nutritional EFA products hit the market. Since then, other health benefits have also been discovered.

The exact mechanism involved in the metabolism of EFAs is not yet understood. The balance among EFAs in the body is crucial. An experienced practitioner can recommend the foods and supplements needed to achieve such balance. Omega-3 EFAs are currently being evaluated at the New York University Child Study Center as a treatment for chronic tic disorders and TS in children and teens. The study is in its second year of funding by the Tourette Syndrome Association and was still in progress as this book went to press (2005). Participants are receiving supplementation with either fish oil or olive oil (the placebo). Lead researcher, Vilma Gabbay, MD, with Barbara J. Coffey, MD and Carmen Alonso, MD, hypothesize that omega-3 EFA supplements will reduce tics and obsessive-compulsive symptoms in this group by affecting serotonin action. Dr. Gabbay told us that she initially applied for the research grant because patients had reported a reduction in tics in their children during the use of omega-3 supplements.

> The exact mechanism involved in the metabolism of essential fatty acids is not yet understood. The balance among EFAs in the body is crucial. An experienced practitioner can recommend the foods and supplements needed to achieve such balance.

Determining needs for essential fatty acids

A red blood cell analysis is considered by some experts to be one of the best methods of measuring fatty acid levels to determine whether specific supplementation is needed. A few laboratories that offer this analysis are listed on the following page.

William J. Walsh, PhD, explained for ACN: "We have had considerable success in using polyunsaturated fatty acids to treat persons with mental illness but have also found that omega-3 and omega-6 oils can cause a worsening of symptoms if given inappropriately. The ideal treatment scenario would be to identify a person's biochemical individuality with respect to polyunsaturated fatty acids, then treat accordingly."

On the other hand, some specialists suggest that the cost of laboratory testing for EFA levels can be avoided by conducting trials of supplementation and carefully observing symptoms. Reports to ACN document that use of fish oil helps reduce tics for some people, yet others find it can aggravate symptoms; they may need a different type of fatty acid (such as from flaxseed or walnuts) or they may not need any supplementation.

Potential adverse side effects associated with the use of fish oil, especially in large doses, include mania, blood thinning, and changes in blood sugar levels. Essential fatty acid supplements can also interact with medications. Check with your doctor before using.

Laboratories can assess essential fatty acid status through a red blood cell analysis. Testing for "free fatty acids" is not the same thing and will not provide the information required. These sites presently perform this analysis and can be shared with your physician:

MetaMetrix: *www.metrametrix.com*; Genova Diagnostics: *www.genovadx.com*; BioCenter: *www.biocenterlab.com*

Finding quality EFA sources

Essential fatty acid plant sources include dark green leafy vegetables and soy bean products. Evening primrose, borage, flaxseed, black currant seed, peanut, walnut, soy, olive, and canola oil are also good sources of EFAs. Fish oil is the most abundant source of omega-3. Some fish oils contain elevated levels of mercury or other contaminants as a result of pollution. Therefore, it is important to find a pure source. Essential fatty acid products must also be fresh; flax and some other oils need refrigeration. Thus, routinely note the freshness date stamped on the container, and look for oils that have been processed at low temperatures.

Docosahexaenoic acid (DHA), one of the most beneficial nutrients in fish oil, is now available from a vegetarian source, algae: Neuromins DHA (see *www.dhadepot.com*).

Vitamin E and tardive dyskinesia

Tardive dyskinesia is a devastating chronic disorder of the nervous system that can develop from extended therapy with some drugs used for tic disorders. In other words, in an attempt to treat one movement disorder, another one is created. Symptoms of tardive dyskinesia include involuntary, and sometimes permanent, jerky movements of the face, tongue, jaws, trunk, and limbs. Older antipsychotic drugs, such as haloperidol (Haldol), pimozide (Orap), and fluphenazine (Prolixin), are most likely to cause the problem, but even some of the newer medications are not without risk. Preliminary reports that vitamin E supplementation can help improve the condition are encouraging, although results are mixed. Additional research suggests that using vitamin E along with vitamin C may reduce existing symptoms. Other antioxidants are currently being researched.

More studies are needed, however, to clarify benefits of nutritional supplementation in the prevention and treatment of tardive dyskinesia.

Biologic categories or subgroups

In the 1970s, William J. Walsh, PhD, completed a study on 24 sets of brothers at the Pfeiffer Treatment Center in Warrenville, Illinois. One brother in each set had symptoms that were diagnosed as TS. Dr. Walsh and his team found that those in the study with TS had a range of chemical imbalances, including one group with unusual trace metal patterns. The researchers concluded that TS is not a single condition. Rather, there are individual "phenotypes" (biologic makeups) that may require completely different treatment approaches. Dr. Walsh explained that the results of his study are preliminary and dated, and they do not allow for specific categorization of these subgroups. Since that time, scientific advances have been made in assessment techniques and analysis. Additional research in this area would be valuable.

> Dr. Walsh and his team found that those in the study with TS had a range of chemical imbalances, including one group with unusual trace metal patterns. The researchers concluded that TS is not a single condition.

Dr. Walsh's work in the area of nutritional factors for depression is a useful model for understanding how defining biological subgroups for tic disorders could be beneficial. The subgroups are also of interest to the many people with tic disorders who also experience depression. After analyzing laboratory data for more than 3,000 clients with clinical depression, Dr. Walsh shared the following insights with ACN, describing five categories of depression profiles that may direct treatment:

Hypercupremia (elevated copper): This condition is especially prevalent in women who experience postpartum and other forms of hormonal depression. Treatment responds well to nutrient therapy and focuses on promoting the metallothionein protein system to achieve a proper balance of trace metals.

Undermethylated (high histamine): These patients often have addictive or obsessive-compulsive perfectionism. They tend to have allergy and seasonal onset of depression. Use of SAMe and a number of other nutrients can be beneficial.

Overmethylated: These patients usually exhibit a combination of anxiety and depression, and are prone to panic attacks. Recommended treatment centers on nutrient therapy aimed at reducing dopamine and norepinephrine levels.

Toxicity: A small percentage of depressive patients exhibit heavy-metal or organic toxicity as their primary chemical imbalance.

Pyrrole disorders: This chemical imbalance is associated with depression, high anxiety, and poor stress control. Pyrroluria is a feature of many behavior and emotional disorders. It is an inborn error of pyrrole chemistry that results in a dramatic deficiency of zinc, vitamin B_6, and arachidonic acid. B_6 is a cofactor for serotonin. Common symptoms include explosive temper, emotional mood swings, poor short-term memory, and frequent infections. The decisive laboratory test is an analysis for kryptopyrroles in urine. Treatment is centered on zinc and B_6 supplements together with omega-6 essential fatty acids.

A similar identification of subgroups for tic disorders would help in the development of appropriate nutritional treatment plans. Dr. Walsh has indicated an interest in pursuing such research, should funding be available.

Calming ADHD with nutrients

We know that many children with tics also have attention deficit hyperactivity disorder (ADHD). We can learn from numerous studies that examine the effect of nutrition on ADHD, and these efforts can point the way for the type of research that needs to be completed for tics and TS. For example, a recent published report indicates that those with ADHD also frequently have an iron deficiency. The more severe the deficiency, the more serious the ADHD symptoms. Low magnesium levels have also been linked to attention deficit disorders, and supplementing with magnesium has improved symptoms; zinc has also been determined to be a key player. Additional nutrients studied and shown helpful for ADHD are the B vitamins and C, essential fatty acids and select amino acids (eg, carnitine), and pycnogenol (an antioxidant usually extracted from pine bark) and grapeseed extract.

A comprehensive nutritional plan for ADHD has recently been found to be as effective as methylphenidate (Ritalin), without the associated adverse effects. The treatment by lead researcher, Karen L. Harding, PhD, included more than fifty nutrients in balanced formula preparations. Similar nutritional efforts can be helpful for ADD—attentional difficulties without hyperactive behaviors.

Combination nutrient products

It is ideal to have professional advice on nutrient therapy, yet many people cannot afford the cost of repeated office visits and laboratory tests—many of which are not covered by insurance. To complicate matters, even when finances are not a problem, it is not easy to find a suitably trained and skilled practitioner.

> Families may turn to combination products for brain support. These supplements contain multiple nutrients—the same concept as the daily multivitamin. This can sometimes be helpful, to varying degrees.

Because of these and other challenges, families may turn to combination products for brain support. These supplements contain multiple nutrients—the same concept as the daily multivitamin. This can sometimes be helpful, to varying degrees. The concern always exists that some of the nutrients could contribute to an imbalance in the body, depending on one's biochemical makeup.

EMPowerplus (Essential Mineral Power Plus), developed by TrueHope Nutritional Support, Ltd., a Canadian-based nonprofit organization in Raymond, Alberta, includes vitamins, antioxidants, and amino acids. Four independent studies support its effectiveness in one or more conditions difficult to treat with conventional medicine: bipolar disorder, behavior disorders, explosive rage, and anxiety. The studies are encouraging, though small. More information is available at: *www.truehope.com*.

Bontech supplement products were developed by Bonnie Grimaldi for patients with TS, ADHD, and OCD. The program she suggests involves supplements along with dietary changes. ACN has received numerous anecdotal reports that Grimaldi's program has helped to significantly reduce tic symptoms in some cases. At this point, there is no way to predict the percentage of people using Bontech Supplements, Ltd, products who may benefit, nor what role recommended dietary adjustments have in improving symptoms versus supplements alone. Details are available at: *www.bonniegr.com*.

David Perlmutter, MD, director of the Perlmutter Health Center in Naples, Florida, has earned a reputation for innovative scientific research. A medical writer and neurologist in private practice, he has developed nutrient products for general brain support:

Brain Sustain, Brain Sustain Neuroactives, and Kids Brain Sustain. Details are available at *www.perlhealth.com.*

Editor's note: ACN does not benefit financially from the sale of any supplements, nor is it endorsing any products discussed here. There are other related products on the market as well. If any adverse effects are noted, discontinue use and inform your practitioner.

Herbal therapy

Kava: This herb is known to be beneficial in relieving symptoms of stress and helpful in promoting sleep. Concerns arose in the 1990s that kava supplements might cause liver dysfunction which resulted in the supplement being banned in several countries. A team of University of Hawaii scientists has suggested that the problem emerged when the demand for the herb increased dramatically. Apparently, in response, manufacturers in Europe adulterated the capsules with bark peelings which are normally discarded. These peelings contain a substance that has a negative effect on the liver. Recently, the use of kava supplements has started to climb again. However, it is important to check with your health practitioner for advice on kava and closely monitor the herb's use.

Valerian: Valerian has long been considered a muscle and nerve relaxant, and a sleep aid. It is considered safe, without known adverse effects, yet long-term use has not been evaluated. Despite its popularity, research is mixed on valerian as a sleep aid.

Bacopa (Bacopa Monnieri): Also known as brahmi, bacopa has been proven to improve brain cell activity and provide a tranquilizing effect. Research indicates that it has anti-stress and antidepressant qualities It is also reported to boost mental acuity and make learning new information easier. No adverse effects are reported, but long-term use has not been fully evaluated.

Spearmint and chamomile teas: Both of these herbs are known for their relaxing properties.

Passiflora incarnata: This herb from the passion flower family has been shown in numerous studies to play a supportive role in inducing sleep. It is also used as an anti-spasmodic.

Down the Hatch!

School-aged kids and even adults can be resistant to swallowing supplements. It is especially difficult to get children to take medication or supplements. It can take cajoling and imagination, but when your child needs them, it is important to make the effort. You can adapt the following suggestions for all ages.

When the child can't swallow tablets, pills, or capsules:

- Find out whether the nutrient is available in a liquid, sublingual (placed under the tongue), or powder.

- Crush or chop the tablet or pill—or empty the capsule if needed. Check supplement instructions first to make sure this is all right to do. Some supplements may need to be taken whole. For those that do not, pill splitters are available at drug stores.

- Mix capsule contents, or the crushed tablet with a few tablespoons of applesauce, pudding, yogurt, mashed potato, mashed banana, frozen raspberry juice concentrate, etc. You might want to occasionally use a small amount of natural fruit sorbet or ice cream (soy and rice substitutes are available for those avoiding milk). The key here is to use a small amount. If the serving is too large, it might not be completely eaten, and therefore the correct amount of the nutrient won't have been taken. Encourage the child to swallow quickly and avoid chewing.

- Blend nutrients into a small smoothie but only when nutrients are not strongly flavored.

- Mix powders with a little sugar (if tolerated), stevia, honey, or dry natural fruit-drink powder. Place on a bit of bread and fold over. After this is eaten, follow with liquid.

- Try putting the supplement in the mouth, taking a sip of liquid then dropping the head down before swallowing. It seems as though it wouldn't help—but it can!

- Use a straw instead of taking a sip of water from a glass; put the medicine in the mouth, then drink from the straw. This can help in the swallowing process.

When giving liquid supplements:

- When using a dropper, place it on the side of the tongue, partway back. Anything placed right in the center of the tongue could cause gagging.

- Use an oral syringe (with no needle, of course), and squirt near the back of the tongue, on the side.

- Chill liquid supplements; cold helps dull the sensation of taste.

If a serious swallowing problem continues, seek professional advice.

Extracts of Ginseng* (Panax quinquefolium) *and Gingko biloba: Both have been shown in a preliminary study to improve symptoms of ADHD.

Combination herbal preparations: Products developed by natural health expert Andrew T. Weil, MD, (*www.askdrweil.com*) and the Life Extension Foundation (*www.lef.org*) are said to reduce stress and relax the body; we did not locate studies on these products.

If you wish to begin herbal therapy in supplement form or in teas, be sure to seek out reputable sources to avoid harmful contaminants from unreliable companies and heed the following caution:

A note of caution

As a general rule, natural substances are much safer than most prescription medications. This does not mean they cannot produce adverse effects or that they can safely be taken indiscriminately. (Avoid the temptation to assume that if one is good, two must be better.) Educate yourself on potential side effects. It is best to consult with practitioners experienced in nutritional and herbal therapy who can guide you. Some nutrients and herbs can interact with each other, or with medications, so you should inform your prescribing physician about any supplements you intend to take or are already taking.

> As a general rule, natural substances are much safer than most prescription medications. This does not mean they cannot produce adverse effects.

Select high-quality brands, monitor symptoms closely, and stop or reduce the dosage of any that seem to be linked to an adverse effect. With some nutrients, symptoms may worsen for a week or two before they improve. Expert advice can help you avoid discontinuing a potentially beneficial supplement prematurely.

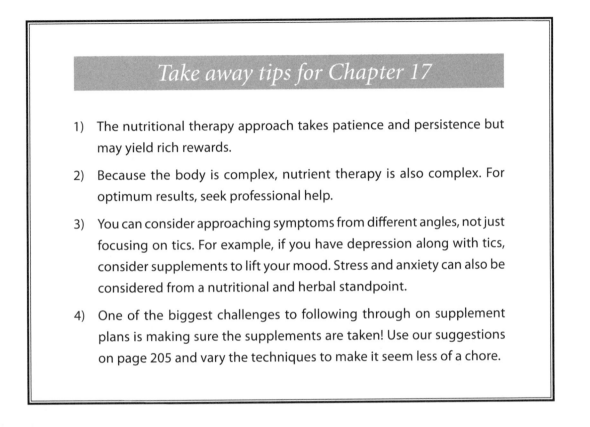

Take away tips for Chapter 17

1) The nutritional therapy approach takes patience and persistence but may yield rich rewards.

2) Because the body is complex, nutrient therapy is also complex. For optimum results, seek professional help.

3) You can consider approaching symptoms from different angles, not just focusing on tics. For example, if you have depression along with tics, consider supplements to lift your mood. Stress and anxiety can also be considered from a nutritional and herbal standpoint.

4) One of the biggest challenges to following through on supplement plans is making sure the supplements are taken! Use our suggestions on page 205 and vary the techniques to make it seem less of a chore.

Notes:

_____

_____

_____

_____

_____

_____

SECTION SIX

Clinical and Research Insights

CHAPTER

18

Identifying and Treating *Candida Albicans*-Related Problems

Interviews with William G. Crook, MD, and William Shaw, PhD

THE CONCEPT OF CANDIDA ALBICANS CAUSING ILLNESS was controversial when first popularized by Dr. William G. Crook more than two decades ago. How could *Candida albicans (C albicans)*—a family of yeasts that typically lives in the digestive tract, the vagina, and the skin—be responsible for fatigue, brain fog and difficulty concentrating, as well as aches and pains, depression, and numerous other disorders? Although blasted by his critics, Dr. Crook continued in his mission to inform the public of what he considered a major health problem. He also shared ways to manage *C albicans* after compiling advice from physicians and patients around the world until his death in 2002. Management included a sugar-free diet, avoidance of fermented foods, and antiyeast medication if warranted; research increasingly supports Dr. Crook's premise.

This chapter contains technical material.

Heiko Santelmann, MD, of Norway has pursued compelling studies on *C albicans*. His most recent work, published in January 2005, focuses on *C albicans* and irritable bowel syndrome, but also includes an excellent review of the possible role of *C albicans* and other yeasts in illness. He links *C albicans* to idiopathic (arising from an unknown source) food intolerances as well as to chemical sensitivities and reduced alcohol tolerance, among other conditions.

Millions of patients and many conventional and integrative practitioners now recognize the importance of *C albicans,* and methods for testing its presence in the body continue to improve. William Shaw, PhD, of Great Plains Laboratory, Lenexa, Kansas, is a leader in the development of *C albicans* testing and treatment protocols. An interview with Dr. Shaw is included in this chapter.

An interview with William G. Crook, MD
An Overview of the Yeast Connection

Dr. Crook , author of the best-selling book, The Yeast Connection, *founded the International Health Foundation and was active in exploring the role of* C albicans *in attention deficit disorders. Sheila J. Rogers interviewed Dr. Crook for* Latitudes *approximately two years before his passing in 2002. Excerpts are included below:*

Dr. Crook, what is your opinion of recent studies suggesting that sugar has nothing to do with attention deficit/hyperactivity disorder?

Back in the 1970s, I didn't know why sugar could cause hyperactivity. Now I think I know the answer. In 1979, I learned about the "yeast connection" from C. Orian Truss, MD. *C albicans* is one of many types of yeast. In addition to vaginal yeast overgrowth, a topic most of your readers are familiar with, *C albicans* can grow in both an adult's and a child's digestive tract and cause a disturbance in immune-system functioning. *C albicans* overgrowth in the intestinal tract can also cause what has been called a "leaky gut." Normally, the lining of the intestines provides a barrier that allows only properly digested substances to pass through and enter the bloodstream. When the lining is damaged and compromised, leakage of imperfectly digested substances, such as proteins (peptides) can occur. These substances are presumed by the immune system to be foreign because they are not normally in the bloodstream. This triggers an antibody reaction. More food allergens and toxins are absorbed, and this can result in a variety of symptoms such as fatigue, headache, irritability, depression, and hyperactivity.

Sugars and other simple carbohydrates promote yeast growth. I realized that many of the youngsters I worked with had increased hyperactivity with consumption of sugars (cane sugar, beet sugar, corn sugar, corn syrup), and it occurred to me that the sugars were "feeding" their *C albicans*.

What do you recommend as treatment for these children?

I began to help a number of patients by eliminating sugar from their diets and giving them prescription and nonprescription antiyeast medication. In 1993, researchers at St. Jude's Children's Hospital, Memphis, Tennessee, conducted a study on mice with weakened immune systems. They gave glucose to one group of mice; the control group received a sugar-free diet. The result was that the yeast in the gastrointestinal tract of the group given glucose was 200 times greater than in the control group. Eliminating sugar is an important first step in dietary changes.

Which children are most likely to have this problem?

In *Clinical Pediatrics* (1987), Randi J. Hagerman, MD, and a colleague reported on a study of children with learning and behavior problems. More than 90% of the children medicated for hyperactivity had experienced three or more ear infections, and 69% had more than ten ear infections. In contrast, only 50% of nonhyperactive children with learning problems had three or more infections, and only 20% of this group had more than ten ear infections.

> Repeated rounds of antibiotics given for ear infections set up a cycle that includes repeated infections and increased nervous system symptoms. This cycle occurs because antibiotics destroy bacteria of many types—not only the "enemies."

In my opinion, repeated rounds of antibiotics given for ear infections set up a cycle that includes repeated infections and increased nervous system symptoms. This cycle occurs because antibiotics destroy bacteria of many types—not only the "enemies" for which they were intended but also the "friends" in your digestive tract that help to manage yeast overgrowth. It is suspected that once the balance in the body has been destroyed by the antibiotics, yeast overgrowth is more likely to occur.

As you've seen in the press and media, the use of Ritalin (methylphenidate) is on the rise. An article in *USA Weekend* stated that the production and sale of Ritalin increased ninefold in just ten years. Although Ritalin is a useful medication that can help control the symptoms of ADD and ADHD, the drug doesn't address the factors causing these problems. In my experience, a tremendous number of children with ADHD can be helped by a sugar-free tailored diet and oral antiyeast medication.

Of course, that's not the whole story. It's true that some children need and will benefit from Ritalin, preferably in conjunction with some of the suggestions I've offered. And there are cases where the best diet management or nutritional support is not enough to correct the problem. Parents should not feel guilty when it is necessary to resort to Ritalin or a similar medication. By following the strategy I've outlined, parents can frequently reduce the amount of medication that may be needed in those cases.

What are the antiyeast medications you might recommend?

Let's look at the two categories: prescription and nonprescription approaches. Non-prescription treatments that can help control *C albicans* overgrowth and restore normal bacteria in the intestinal tract include caprylic acid, probiotics (such as preparations of *lactobacillus acidophilus* and other friendly probiotic bacteria), citrus seed extracts (sold as Paracan 144, Paramicrocidin, and Citricidal), garlic cloves and/or Kyolic, and the herbal product, Mathake (*Teriminalia catappa*). The management program should be directed by a physician, although it is not always easy to locate a doctor who is well-versed in the subject.

Prescription drugs can also be useful. These primarily include nystatin, Diflucan, Sporanox, and Nizoral.

You said earlier that control of diet and antiyeast medications were not the "whole story". What else should our readers be aware of in order to gain control?

Nutritional supplements can be very important. Look for yeast-free, sugar-free, color-free multivitamins, minerals, and antioxidant preparations. Children with ADHD may also benefit from essential fatty acids; I recommend flaxseed oil. It's very safe and has both the omega-3 and omega-6 fatty acids. It can be used in salad dressing or taken as a straight supplement. However, it's important that it be fresh. I also recommend grapeseed extract and pycnogenol (from pine bark).

Before embarking on a yeast management program, one should rule out allergies to dust, molds, and inhalants, as these can also affect nervous system functioning. People with yeast-related health problems are almost always overly sensitive to everyday chemicals in the environment. Therefore, try to eliminate use of perfumes, carpet odors, cleaning products, paints, insecticides, tobacco smoke, diesel fumes, etc. In regard to diet, it's best to purchase organic foods and to choose prepared foods in glass containers rather than plastic. Additional dietary recommendations are included in my books.

Parents should encourage the hyperactive child to spend less time in front of the TV and more time outside in clean air. Of course, love, encouragement, praise, laughter, and lots of hugs are important too.

An interview with William Shaw, PhD
Identifying Candida albicans *problems*

Dr. Shaw is an expert and frequent lecturer on nutritional biochemistry and laboratory medicine. His most recent book is Biological Treatments for Autism and PDD *(Pervasive Developmental Delay). Perhaps most recognized for his work with autism, he has also demonstrated a special interest in tic disorders. Dr. Shaw has board-certifications in both clinical chemistry and toxicology. He is a past associate professor at the University of Missouri at the Kansas City School of Medicine and served as director of clinical chemistry, toxicology, and endocrinology at Children's Mercy Hospital, Kansas City, Missouri. Dr. Shaw is now the director of The Great Plains Laboratory in Lenexa, Kansas. This interview is by Sheila J. Rogers.*

Would you please talk about the role of Candida albicans *in neuropsychiatric conditions?*

As you have discussed in *Latitudes*, many people with attention deficit disorders and hyperactivity, Tourette syndrome, autism, depression, obsessive-compulsive disorder (OCD), and other neuropsychiatric conditions report food sensitivities. *C albicans* is one of the most common disease-causing species of yeast, and it can play a key role in biochemic pathways that involve the central nervous system.

Yeast can exist in two forms: as a floating single cell or as a colony form. In the colony form, yeast secrete enzymes, such as *phospholipase*, and *proteases* that break down the lining of the intestinal tract allowing the yeast colony to attach to the intestinal wall. This results in holes in the intestinal wall, referred to as *leaky gut syndrome*. In this syndrome, large undigested food molecules that would normally be blocked and broken down instead pass through the lining and are absorbed into the bloodstream; this then elicits food allergies. Neurologic reactions have been associated with these food allergies, thus, healing the leaky gut can reduce food sensitivities for many people.

How do you recommend people test for the presence of C albicans?

Let's first look at testing for yeast in the gastrointestinal tract. The most common test is stool testing, and this can be very useful. There are conditions, however, under which the stool test gives false-negative results and a yeast problem is not identified. An example is the condition in which the patient has a high IgA—the antibody in the nasal passages and gastrointestinal lining that protects from germs. It is secreted by Peyers' patches, the part of the immune system that surrounds the gastrointestinal tract.

There are some cases where symptoms suggest an overgrowth of *C albicans* in the intestine, yet when a stool specimen is cultured in Petri dishes, the presence of the yeast is not indicated. In these cases, often when we measure the IgA in the stool, it's extremely high. In such cases, we often also find high amounts of yeast by-products by using a different test. This test is based on the principle that there are fermentation products of the yeast that are formed in the intestinal tract and then are absorbed from the intestine and passed into the circulatory system—the blood vessels surrounding the intestine. From there, the products proceed and *C albicans* by-products are then distributed to the rest of the body. When that blood is filtered, those same by-products can be measured. We use a urine test at The Great Plains Laboratory, called the *Organic Acid Test*, not for detecting *C albicans* in urine, but to detect these by-products which reveal the presence of yeast in the gastrointestinal tract.

We have found in many cases that these fermentation products were notably high with a corresponding high IgA. It can also happen that the yeast are not in the lumen of the intestine, but instead burrowed into the lining of the gastrointestinal tract. In these cases, the stool analysis may show a negative result and yet the yeast are present.

As far as blood tests, you can measure yeast by-products, and you can do yeast cultures. Such cultures are usually negative unless the person is extremely ill because a large number are required for positive results. There is also a new technology available for blood testing, called the *Polymerase Chain Reaction* (PCR), in which the nucleic acid of the yeast is measured. We have used this technology for many cases even when the yeast culture in the blood is negative. The PCR is more sensitive and will actually detect *C albicans* in measurable amounts in the blood.

> It can also happen that the yeast are not in the lumen of the intestine, but instead burrowed into the lining of the gastrointestinal tract. In these cases, the stool analysis may show a negative result, and yet the yeast are present.

Isn't it true that there is still considerable controversy about the role of C albicans —with many conventional practitioners refuting the concept that it could affect brain function?

Many people have a difficult time seeing why gastrointestinal yeast should have neurotoxic effects, but I think it's very clear that the by-products of yeast can have significant toxicity for the body. For example, gliotoxins are small, molecular-weight compounds that impair the immune system and actually kill white blood cells. This is one of the reasons why people with *C albicans* have problems with recurrence; it is because their immune system has been impaired by the strains of the yeast that produce the gliotoxin. Not all *C albicans* produce these, but nearly 50% of the strains do. This aspect has not been addressed sufficiently by the medical community, and some mainstream physicians will dismiss the fact that intestinal yeast can cause central nervous system problems. But they are ignoring the issue of these small molecular-weight compounds that can be extremely toxic. It is estimated that just 1 milligram of this gliotoxin (an amount equal to a grain of salt) can be fatal. It's comparable to *botulinum toxin*, which also can act as a lethal type of toxin.

In addition, *C albicans* yeast can produce many other by-products, such as a sugar called *arabinose,* which has the ability to cross-link proteins of many different types. The place where the yeast cross-links these proteins is a critical part of the molecule that most frequently is the active part of the protein. The arabinose from yeast has the ability to react with these active sites of the proteins and thereby deactivate their biochemic function, which can be enzymatic. The function could be involved in transport or in assisting with the action of vitamins; it could be acting as a binding protein. All of these functions can potentially be impaired by this cross-linking action of the arabinose.

The proteins that would be most susceptible are those that have high levels of two specific amino acids with which this yeast by-product reacts. These two amino acids are *arginine* and *lysine*. The *C albicans* actually forms a cross-linkage between lysine and arginine. The proteins in the body that are most rich in these proteins and the most susceptible are the *histones*. These proteins are important because they are present in the nucleus, and they are involved with the regulation of the genes: whether the gene is turned off or on. When a small child between, let's say, six months and two or three years of age, has high amounts of these by-products, it could significantly alter the pattern of the regulation of the histones, resulting in abnormal development. This is a way in which a simple by-product of *C albicans*—a simple sugar which is ordinarily not found in human metabolism—can cause a significant problem.

Arabinose is not typically found in human metabolism?

Right. In other words, humans do not normally produce this sugar. In addition, the arabinose blocks the three important sites where vitamins B$_6$, biotin, and lipoic acid function. All of these are important in a number of oxidation reduction reactions in the cell. These are important coenzymes that are probably involved in close to a hundred biochemic reactions that are important to human biochemistry.

In what other conditions do you see a connection with C albicans, particularly with children?

In children, we see this commonly in ADD and ADHD—perhaps even higher than in those with autism. I would say we have seen this connection in perhaps 90% of the attention deficit disorder/hyperactivity cases with which we have been involved. We also see it commonly in children with seizure disorders, and I think that's the reason the ketogenic diet, or the simple carbohydrate diet, has been successful for some seizure conditions. Many people are familiar with this diet, which is almost completely carbohydrate-restricted. I suspect one reason the diet is effective may be because it is essentially an antiyeast diet. The antiyeast diet is called a "caveman" diet in which most carbohydrates are severely restricted, especially in the first couple of months of treatment. And because the incidence of yeast is so high in many children with seizure disorders, I suspect that it may play a major role in the cause of some seizures.

We also have had experience with a number of children with Tourette syndrome and often find a high incidence of *C albicans* here as well. Treatment of *dysbiosis*—the condition of living with intestinal flora that has harmful effects—can improve Tourette symptoms in some cases. We see that a yeast problem can affect a wide range of children's neuropsychiatric, or neurodevelopmental diseases, as well as schizophrenia in adults.

There is another side effect of the yeast; it produces certain compounds called *cyclic peptides* that inhibit one of the key regulators of our hormonal system. The enzyme is *DPP4*, which is involved in regulating either the activation or deactivation of approximately 30 or 40 peptide hormones. So when this enzyme is knocked out by a yeast inhibitor, which is found in great amounts in *C albicans*, there can be a disruption of the hormonal system. This enzyme is also involved in regulating digestion and in regulating a number of immune modulators, the *cytokines*. All of these can be affected by a simple low-molecular weight compound which is readily absorbed from the gastrointestinal tract.

> There is another side effect of the yeast; it produces certain compounds called cyclic peptides that inhibit one of the key regulators of our hormonal system.

So, even in the case where the yeast has not invaded the bloodstream and the rest of the body, it can have marked effects from these different toxic compounds that are produced by *C albicans*.

What are your recommendations for antiyeast treatment?

The most critical thing to remember is that in some conditions, the problem with *C albicans* is severe. A lot of people don't realize that *C albicans* management has to be long-term. We see this especially in children with autism in which case *C albicans* seems to be more severe than in other conditions. In some cases, I would recommend treatment for at least one year with nystatin or other appropriate drugs. There's a wide range of drugs that are effective including over-the-counter herbal remedies. My experience is that all of these can be effective, to some degree, and indeed I've received reports of all of them being effective in various cases. But it depends on the particular sensitivity. So the test that we usually recommend to pinpoint problem areas is the one that combines testing the by-products of the yeast and the stool testing. By doing both of these, you greatly increase the chance of finding the yeast. If the yeast can be cultured from the stool test—which, I have explained, does not always occur—you can pinpoint the agents that will be most specific in treating it.

When the stool test doesn't specify the types of yeast involved, should people then just pursue therapeutic trial and error?

Right. They can do trial and error, and they can assess its success on the clinical response. However, note that there is often an initial die-off reaction, which can temporarily increase symptoms. This, in fact, is an indication that the program is effective.

For autism, I would estimate that between 30% and 40% of children have the by-products of *Clostridia*, a bacteria, and roughly between 60% to 70% have a problem with *C albicans*. The control of *Clostridia* has been effective in managing some cases of tic disorders, as well. In one case, probiotics eliminated tics after just a few days of treatment.

How does this tie-in to dietary recommendations?

It's known that the two foods that are the greatest issue in autism, as well as in attention deficit disorders, are peptides from wheat and milk. We see preliminary evidence that there's a *C albicans* peptide as well; we suspect that it has a similar structure to the peptides from wheat and milk, and so it has the same opiate effect. This is why the symptoms can be notably similar with any of these sensitivities, whether it's the wheat, milk or the *C albicans*, because they may be affecting the same receptor sites. Recent work has confirmed that *C albicans* has a cell wall protein in which 150 amino acids are identical to those in gluten.

When you say "we see" are you talking about doctors who have referred laboratory work to you, or do you oversee a clinic?

We get feedback from both physicians and parents. We also have an associated clinic. When the family doesn't have a physician who is actively involved in the case, we can provide advice and they can try, let's say, herbal treatments. We get feedback in that way. Sometimes the family's physician is willing to order a test but isn't willing to go along with the treatment based on the testing. In these cases, we can offer information on select herbal remedies that families can try. We have a trained nutritional consultant available to give advice, and that's included in the price of the testing.

What tests do you recommend for classic tic conditions including Tourette syndrome?

In addition to *C albicans* testing, doctors often screen for IgG food allergies and heavy metals. This includes the blood heavy metals test. We often initially do a hair test because it has high sensitivity, and it is easy to collect the sample. It's not perfect, and when a person had the exposure to a metal many years before, the test might not indicate its presence, but I'd say that's my favorite test when you're only going to perform one test.

When you want to be more thorough, you could also do a blood test for heavy metals at the same time. Additional laboratory work, including testing of urine amino acids, might also be useful in certain cases.

Would you please describe your food sensitivity test compared with other types of food allergy or sensitivity testing?

Well, this is an area of controversy. I want to say that right up front. We have found that the IgG food allergy testing is the most appropriate and useful for those individuals with developmental issues or neuropsychiatric conditions. Several scientific articles have documented the benefits of IgG tests. We found large numbers of people who were tested using the traditional allergy test (RAST) and the IgE results often came back as negative; therefore, we received little useful information. We recognize that the American Academy of Allergy, Asthma and Immunology (Milwaukee, Wisconsin) recommends IgE testing, but they are focused on classic allergy. We're looking at something different. We are focused on antibodies that may cross-react with the blood-brain barrier. These antibodies are causing reactions that we don't understand completely, but we've found that clinically, they are extremely useful. We've learned that when you come up with a positive value that's high and you eliminate that problem food, you're frequently going to achieve good results. The most common food allergies by far are milk and wheat, and these allergies occur in a wide range of conditions. I often recommend that milk and wheat be eliminated on a trial basis. The IgE test is more useful for the inhalant allergies, such as dust, mold, mildew, cats and dogs—that type of thing. We offer inhalant allergy testing; sometimes those allergic reactions will be triggers for tics.

Do you have any theory as to why C albicans *currently appears to be such a widespread problem?*

There are some possible tie-ins with the evidence for vaccine damage. For example, mercury (thimerosal) has just recently been removed from most vaccines. Mercury specifically inhibits enzymes in white blood cells, including a particular one called *myeloperoxidase* which is used by the cells to kill *C albicans*. This is one way thimerosal in vaccines may be involved in recurrent *C albicans*. Though *C albicans* and vaccines may seem like entirely different issues, they may be related.

In addition, the measles virus causes recurrent Candidiasis when given to animals. A recent article reported that the measles vaccine severely depressed cellular immunity to *C albicans* in 85% of children tested. So both the virus itself, or the particular vaccine strain of the virus, as well as the mercury in the vaccine may play a role in recurrent *C albicans* which is, as I mentioned, one of the most difficult issues in treating autism. It's also possible that when children are given multiple vaccines on the same day this may be more detrimental to the immune system than if the inoculations had been spread out.

> A recent article reported that the measles vaccine severely depressed cellular immunity to *C albicans* in 85% of children tested. So both the virus itself, or the particular vaccine strain of the virus, as well as the mercury in the vaccine may play a role in recurrent *C albicans*.

One of the worst risk factors associated with having an adverse reaction to vaccines is whether the child is taking a course of antibiotics at the time of receiving the vaccine. In our experience, this can result in a severe yeast problem because the antibiotic sets the stage, and then the additional viruses and preservatives can, given certain circumstances, depress immunity further. This results in a virulent form of *C albicans* that is much more difficult to control.

What is your professional advice regarding testing for nutrients that are clinically proving to be beneficial for tic disorders, such as magnesium and essential fatty acids?

I agree that these are important nutrients, and deficiencies in these are common. Magnesium deficiency is fairly difficult to access through laboratory testing. My advice would be that you probably don't need testing for it, you can just give it and observe response. The same could be said for essential fatty acids. There is testing available for that, but my own point of view is that you can do a therapeutic trial for one month or so and see whether it has helped. When it helps, keep doing it. When it doesn't help or when symptoms worsen, stop that treatment.

Calcium and magnesium supplementation are readily recommended because deficiencies in these are common, especially in people who have to restrict milk in the diet. We often recommend 1,000 mg a day of calcium from age two years to adult. A liquid can provide the best absorption. When a person is not digesting well, they may be deficient in different nutrients even when the diet is adequate. In a person who's not digesting well, the pill can go in one end and out the other without ever being absorbed. Therefore, the liquid form of calcium might be best, or when liquid is not available, perhaps a chewable calcium supplement.

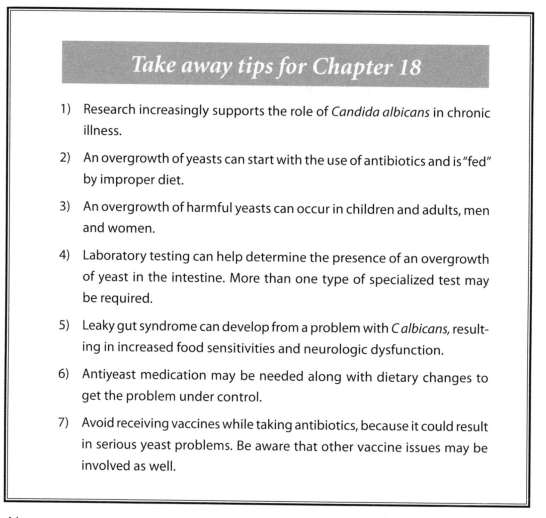

Take away tips for Chapter 18

1) Research increasingly supports the role of *Candida albicans* in chronic illness.

2) An overgrowth of yeasts can start with the use of antibiotics and is "fed" by improper diet.

3) An overgrowth of harmful yeasts can occur in children and adults, men and women.

4) Laboratory testing can help determine the presence of an overgrowth of yeast in the intestine. More than one type of specialized test may be required.

5) Leaky gut syndrome can develop from a problem with *C albicans,* resulting in increased food sensitivities and neurologic dysfunction.

6) Antiyeast medication may be needed along with dietary changes to get the problem under control.

7) Avoid receiving vaccines while taking antibiotics, because it could result in serious yeast problems. Be aware that other vaccine issues may be involved as well.

Notes:

_____

_____

_____

_____

Clinical Laboratory Tests as Treatment Guidance

Jon B. Pangborn, PhD, FAIC, CCN

Editor: A critical aspect of the new mindset needed to successfully treat tic disorders focuses on determining the causes of symptoms. Identifying biologic imbalances that may be affecting the brain is a vital step, and laboratory tests can often accomplish such identification. All those discussed will not be needed for every case, and other additional tests may be recommended when clinically indicated.

This chapter contains technical material.

Dr. Pangborn holds a PhD in chemical engineering, with a background in biochemistry and the field of human metabolism. He is president and founder of Bionostics of St. Charles, Illinois, which provides information to health professionals on metabolism, nutrition, and toxicity. Dr. Pangborn is a fellow of the American Institute of Chemists, an adjunct professor of nutritional biochemistry (The Union Institute, Cincinnati, Ohio), a certified clinical nutritionist, past president of Doctor's Data Laboratory (1988 to 1995), and former consultant on metabolic laboratory tests (Great Smokies Diagnostic Laboratory, 1996 to 2002). He is the author or coauthor of nine United States issued patents, and an international speaker. Dr. Pangborn is a cofounder of the Defeat Autism Now effort and is coauthor of Autism: Effective Biomedical Treatments *(2005) on biomedical options for assessing and treating autistic-spectrum conditions.*

Dr. Jon Pangborn:

TOURETTE SYNDROME FEATURES VARIOUS DEGREES of muscular tics and twitches, often accompanied by inappropriate vocal utterances. It is classified as an extrapyramidal neurologic disorder. Cases vary widely in the extent of such tics and vocal utterances. Many clinicians attribute this to acquired stressors that are added onto a possible genetic predisposition. The laboratory tests outlined here are intended to uncover both the genetic predisposition and the environmental, infectious, or dietary factors that may trigger or worsen the condition.

Tourette syndrome is often linked to an abnormality on the long arm of chromosome 18 at site 18q22.1. Inheritance of TS may be autosomal dominant (uncertain), and not all cases of TS are linked to 18q22.1. (*Harrison's Principles of Internal Medicine*, 13th Ed., p. 2208). Despite linking some cases of TS to 18q22.1, no commonly-available genetics test seems to exist for this disease (chromosome or DNA analysis).

Laboratory tests

Blood platelet adrenal catecholamine analysis for dopa, dopamine and related monoamines: Tourette syndrome appears to feature excessive *dopaminergic activity* relative to cholinergic activity. Blood, and especially blood platelets, carry the catecholamines, and excessive blood or platelet dopamine can be a reason for increased dopaminergic activity. Biochemical reasons for elevated dopamine include copper deficiency or ascorbate deficiency; both nutrients assist the dopamine-processing enzyme, dopamine beta-hydroxylase. Other nutrients or agents that indirectly affect dopamine include: S-adenosylmethionine (SAM or SAMe), the enzyme monoamine oxidase ("MAO") and MAO-inhibitors, and magnesium, which activates an important catecholamine-methylating enzyme.

Blood cell mineral analysis: This is for assessment of magnesium status, for the reasons previously described. Additionally, a magnesium deficiency by itself can cause muscular twitches that mimic or add to those of TS. Daily magnesium supplementation, in some cases, can reduce or eliminate muscle twitches.

Blood or urine analysis for active ascorbate (not the oxidized or dehydroascorbate forms): This is suggested for the reasons previously indicated. Ascorbic acid, vitamin C, also potentiates the effects of some antipsychotic drugs, making them more effective at lower doses. This is important for disorders like TS in which cell-receptor binding sites (message-transfer sites) are incorrectly activated. And, high (pharmacologic) doses of ascorbate may, in some cases lessen inappropriate dopamine-mediated behaviors (Rebec GV: *Science* 1985; Jan 227:438-440).

Blood choline assay: Some research findings are consistent with the thesis that increasing a low choline level can improve the excess dopaminergic condition (Wurtman and Wurtman, *Nutrition and the Brain*, vol3, Raven Press, 1979,167; vol 5, 1979;264–68). Choline can be supplemented nutritionally as lecithin. In April 1998, choline became an "official" essential nutrient, as is a vitamin, for humans. (Blusztajn, *Science* Aug 1998:794–95.)

Comprehensive stool analysis including bacteriology and mycology: This is a stool analysis that includes identification of abnormal bacteria and yeast as well as metabolic markers related to digestion. The rationale for this test is that false neurotransmitters may be generated by a combination of maldigestion, malabsorption, and gut bacteria or yeast. Abnormally increased gastrointestinal permeability (tests also available) can provide a pathway for gut-produced neurotransmitters and neurotoxins to enter the body. Use of digestive enzymes and correction of dysbiotic overgrowth in the intestines (caused by use of antibiotics) and probiotics may decrease or eliminate this source of false neurotransmitters.

Food IgG and inhalant allergy testing: This test may be useful for those with food allergies or reactivities. Food allergies probably do not cause TS, but are not uncommon in individuals with this syndrome. Food reactivities can be related to maldigestion, which can be a cause of dysbiotic bowel flora and false neurotransmitters, which may be causative or worsening factors. IgE-mediated reactions are typically prompt and may be obvious without a clinical test. IgG-mediated reactions are typically not prompt and may be virtually impossible to identify with respect to causative foods. So an IgG analysis can be a valuable help in dietary intervention. Additionally, some clinicians have claimed improvement following identification and elimination or desensitization to inhalant allergens, including those of pollen, mold, and fungal sources.

A blood plasma (fasting) or a 24-hour amino acid analysis: This analysis provides levels of amino acid precursors of neurotransmitters, and it suggests when SAM (SAMe) may be deficient via abnormal methionine levels. Rectifying abnormal levels of amino acids may help to correct neurotransmitter imbalances. A 24-hour urine amino acid analysis should include measured levels of some short-chain dietary peptides (anserine, carnosine), which, when excessive, suggest maldigestion and increased gut permeability. By inference from amino acid results, one can also assess the functional activities of vitamins B_6, B_{12}, and folate. It is my experience that, when abnormal, correcting these vitamin activities can improve the Tourette condition.

Suggestions on ordering tests

Ordering these outlined laboratory tests, understanding the results, and taking appropriate remedial action requires the help of your doctor, often with input from the technical staff at the clinical laboratory. These are specialized analyses that require specific testing protocols, and laboratories that offer them should provide all instructions and a test kit with the required submittal materials. Analytical work to diagnose what's wrong at the molecular level (and possibly improve it) is not a do-it-yourself job. A professional nutritionist may be of considerable help in correcting vitamin, mineral, or amino acid deficiencies.

No single laboratory can provide all of the tests discussed here, and multiple laboratories (at least three different ones) are usually needed when all seven of the clinical tests are to be done. We list some laboratories according to types of testing that are offered as of this writing. Most laboratories are willing to discuss specimen requirements, testing protocols and costs. The list is not meant to be restrictive and reflects only this author's experience. Your doctor may be able to order an equivalent test from a laboratory of his/her choice that is not listed.

Adrenal Catecholamine Analysis (You should request the fractionated blood plasma or blood platelet version, not total levels but individual catecholamine levels, to include dopamine.)

Mayo Medical Laboratory—measures in blood plasma (800) 533-1710

Quest Diagnostics—measures in blood plasma, contact your local laboratory in Yellow Pages for instructions.

Vitamin Diagnostics—measures in blood platelets (732) 583-7773

Blood Plasma or 24-Hour Urine Amino Acid Analysis; Vitamin Analysis (vitamin C, choline); Blood Cell (erythrocyte) Mineral Analysis (especially blood cell magnesium). Two or more laboratories may be needed among the following:

Doctor's Data Lab (DDI) (800) 323-2784

Genova Diagnostics (formerly Great Smokies Diagnostic Lab) (800) 522-4762

Mayo Medical Laboratories (800) 533-1710

Vitamin Diagnostics (732) 583-7773

Comprehensive Stool Analysis

Genova Diagnostics (800) 522-4762

Allergy Testing

Alletess Medical Lab (800) 225-5404

Genova Diagnostics (800) 522-4762

ImmunoLabs (800) 231-9197

Immunosciences Lab (800) 950-4686

York Nutritional Labs (888) 751-3388

Editor: Dr. Pangborn intended this as a starting list for tests that may help in providing treatment guidance for TS and other tic disorders. As he points out, the list is not meant to be restrictive in terms of tests or laboratories, and not all will be needed for every person. Additional tests may be recommended by your physician; tests should be ordered on the basis of a physical and environmental evaluation of the patient. This is an emerging field, and ACN looks forward to providing more information on biological assessments for tics and TS in the future.

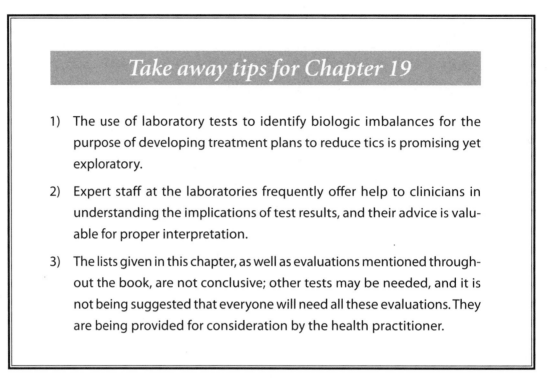

Take away tips for Chapter 19

1) The use of laboratory tests to identify biologic imbalances for the purpose of developing treatment plans to reduce tics is promising yet exploratory.

2) Expert staff at the laboratories frequently offer help to clinicians in understanding the implications of test results, and their advice is valuable for proper interpretation.

3) The lists given in this chapter, as well as evaluations mentioned throughout the book, are not conclusive; other tests may be needed, and it is not being suggested that everyone will need all these evaluations. They are being provided for consideration by the health practitioner.

Notes:

_____

_____

_____

_____

_____

_____

_____

SECTION SEVEN

Additional Therapies

CHAPTER
20

Behavioral and Counseling Therapies

BEHAVIORAL THERAPIES ARE THE ONLY nondrug approaches that have been strictly evaluated for TS and the control of tics. Although limited research suggests that such therapies can be effective for those sufficiently motivated, many patients and doctors are not aware of them, and finding a trained clinician in your area can be difficult.

Habit reversal training

Nathan H. Azrin, PhD, is one of the pioneering researchers in behavioral control of tics, a training that involves learning techniques that can prevent or stop a tic. Dr. Azrin studied with Dr. B. F. Skinner, often denoted as the "father" of behavioral therapy. In an interview with ACN, Dr. Azrin explained that select behavioral therapies can be beneficial for controlling tics when the approach is comprehensive and the practitioner properly trained. This group of techniques is known as *habit reversal training*. Dr. Azrin emphasized that he believes a recent tendency to use a simplified version of the steps he outlined may result in a reduced level of success. Components and variations of habit reversal training are described next, along with other behavioral approaches being used to assist in the control of tics.

Competing response: In this approach, a competing response, or a muscle movement opposite to the movement created by the tic, is used. For example, using isometric tensing of the neck muscles in a downward motion would counter a tic that jerked the head upward. For effective use of a competing response, the opposing muscles are contracted for at least two minutes when an urge to tic arises or a tic has started. The following three components must be part of a competing response:

- It must be opposite to the tic movement;
- It must be capable of being maintained for several minutes;
- It must be socially inconspicuous and easily compatible with normal activities, but incompatible with the tic. For example, when someone has a hand tic, a competing response of sitting on one's hands is not acceptable as this is not socially inconspicuous, and it also interferes with normal activities.

Self-Monitoring: This procedure involves identifying the number of times certain tics occur; for this, a hand-held counter is useful. The goal is to bring about change by developing increased awareness.

Relaxation: Relaxation exercises can include progressive muscle relaxation, visual imagery, deep breathing, and self-statements about the relaxation state. The exercises should be practiced daily to reinforce their effect and can be used whenever there is heightened anxiety or tics. Progressive relaxation is used to release tension throughout the body. This is difficult to do while you are experiencing disruptive tic symptoms. (For simplicity, the reader is addressed as "you" in this discussion although the person needing the relaxation could be a child or someone else.)

Daily practice when you are less symptomatic will help you develop this technique. While lying or sitting, start by becoming aware of the front of your body. Beginning at your feet or your head, gradually and progressively tense and release each muscle area as you move through your body. After you have tensed and released the muscles in the front of your body, move your attention to the back of the body and repeat the process. When you are finished, lie quietly for several minutes. This can be done when alone at work, when riding a bus or train, or while relaxing at home. It is an ideal exercise to do in bed just before sleep.

Deep Breathing: Stress reduction experts suggest becoming more aware of your breathing, and practicing controlled, deep breathing. Practice of these skills will allow you to revert to a relaxed form of breathing during stressful times. Here is a simple exercise to do when you feel the need to calm yourself: Stand up straight then relax your body. Let your arms hang loosely by your side. Close your eyes and imagine that in order to breathe, you must take deep breaths from the soles of your feet. Take several slow breaths in this manner.

Visual imagery: You can do this yourself, with an instructor, or using an audiotape. Close your eyes for several minutes and imagine a relaxing scene or create a mental image of being tic-free. Some people see their body as being filled with a healing light, others project an image of a calm, beautiful lake. Whatever image you choose should elicit a feeling of peace. You may also use affirmative statements to reinforce a sense of calm and counter stressful thoughts. Find the phrases that are most meaningful to you, and couch them in positive terms. Example: Rather than saying or thinking, "I am not anxious or out of control," tell yourself: "I am relaxed and at peace. I am in control."

Contingency management: This is a technique behavioral therapists use to reward a patient for not allowing tics to manifest. A reward can be praise, the promise of an activity, a special treat, money or a particular item. This approach to TS has reportedly been more successful with children than adults. However, the results of studies discourage this technique being used as a single therapy. It is not recommended that parents, teachers, or others try this method with children on their own, as it could have detrimental effects and be emotionally upsetting. Only a professional can determine how contingency management might help as part of a comprehensive behavior-intervention program. It is important for the reader to understand that children and adults cannot readily stop their tics on demand in order to receive a "reward."

Massed negative practice: In this behavioral approach, the adult or child purposefully performs a troublesome tic as quickly and "effortfully" (intentionally, with a feeling of effort) as possible for a designated period—up to 30 minutes, for example—with a rest period at intervals. The idea is to become tired of making the tic.

Hypnosis

Martin H. Young, PhD, director of the Developmental and Behavioral Consultation Program, Worcester, Massachusetts, has been a leader in hypnotherapy for tic disorders. Hypnotherapy in this context does not imply that someone is simply hypnotized in a familiar manner and instructed not to tic anymore. The approach is more complex and requires a disciplined commitment from the person being hypnotized. In 1988, Dr. Young published a treatment method he found successful for children with TS. He combined self-hypnosis with habit reversal and other behavioral techniques, achieving success in a small number of children. Published research indicates a positive outcome in the treatment of TS symptoms by combining hypnotherapy with progressive relaxation, biofeedback, and imagery. Practitioners suggest some people are more suited to this than others; additional study could help define these promising efforts.

Cognitive behavior therapy

Cognitive behavior interventions have been shown to be particularly beneficial for obsessive-compulsive disorder (OCD). In a small number of studies, this technique was also helpful for tic disorders. Cognitive behavior therapy combines cognitive, or thinking techniques, with behavior therapy. By exploring thought processes, the patient is taught to see how certain thinking patterns involved in OCD or anxiety may be responsible for creating a distorted picture of what is actually taking place. A fear that every time we answer the phone, we are going to be told that a loved one has died is an example of distorted or illogical thinking.

> Given the strong connection between mental stress and tics, cognitive behavior therapy is a logical approach for treating tic disorders.

Given the strong connection between mental stress and tics, cognitive behavior therapy is a logical approach for treating tic disorders. Teaching people to be aware of and avoid stressful events or certain social situations that are known to aggravate tics can also be useful. Obstacles to cognitive behavior therapy include finding an experienced therapist and having the discipline to follow through with practice of the technique. Some of the techniques are better suited for adults or older children than young children.

Tamar Chansky, PhD, director of the Children's Center for OCD and Anxiety, Plymouth Meeting, Pennsylvania, has written two books on the use of cognitive behavior therapy and other behavior modification techniques that can reduce OCD symptoms and anxiety. These two conditions often overlap with Tourette syndrome and can add to the psychologic stress associated with TS. These behavior modification treatments may aid people with TS. *Freeing your Child from Obsessive Compulsive Disorder* and *Freeing your Child from Anxiety* are reader-friendly and recommended for parents and practitioners.

Counseling and talk therapy

As in many chronic conditions, emotional issues can play an underlying role in tic disorders. Research, however, does not strongly support talk therapy or psychoanalysis as a singular treatment; counseling by itself should not be expected to eliminate tics. At the same time, it is not unusual for those affected with tics, including TS, to have problems with self-esteem, anger, depression, and coping. Counseling to improve self-acceptance, develop coping skills, or learn how to reduce ongoing stress can help. Education for family members on how to best deal with and support the individual with tics can be very important.

Families often report that when marital problems or other family or social stressors increase, tics also flare. Counseling as a supportive measure to improve the dynamics in the home can have a positive effect.

Meditation and spirituality

As we seek to reduce stress (and thereby reduce tics), meditation is a practical, proven approach. Rajinder Singh, a renowned author on topics of meditation and spirituality, wrote in *Inner and Outer Peace through Meditation*: "Meditation has numerous benefits for our physical and mental well-being. Once we learn how to meditate, we carry within us a ready remedy that we can use at any time and place. . . . Studies show that in meditation, brain waves function at a frequency of 4–10hz. During these states there is a sensation of peace and total relaxation."

Of the meditative practices, transcendental meditation is the most researched for its effect on health. This form of meditation has been proven to decrease psychosocial stress and blood pressure, reduce the use of tobacco and alcohol, and lower high cholesterol.

Similar approaches can also bring benefits. Mindfulness meditation stresses awareness of the moment, a "be here now" mentality that helps release regrets and pains of the past and minimizes fear or anxiety about the future. This can lead to improved responses to anxiety and panic. Research supports the use of mindfulness meditation as a coping mechanism for daily stressors.

Those who are so inclined can find a source of personal strength, courage, and renewal in spirituality. Whether pursued in solitude or in a group setting, through faith in a higher power, people can access this source of refuge and empowerment. Although difficult to quantify, research continues on the efficacy of prayer in a variety of medical and psychologic disorders.

Exercise and yoga

Moderate exercise helps the body detoxify, promotes health, and alleviates stress. Those with tics who excel in or get enjoyment from physical activities, including yoga, may also have improved self-esteem. Unfortunately, some tic symptoms interfere with normal movement and make exercise painful or impossible. Decisions on physical activity have to be made on an individual basis.

The benefit of each activity needs to be weighed against possible trigger situations. Participating in organized sports can be a good social and physical activity, yet the pressure to perform well can be a trigger for increased tic symptoms. There may be times when individual endeavors (yoga, working out, weight-lifting, running) or a game, such as tennis played with a trusted companion, are preferable to team sports.

Swimming is popular, and can be fun and rewarding. At the same time, exposure to the chemicals used in pools can trigger some people's tics. Research has shown that swimming in indoor pools can increase the risk of asthma and other allergic disease. The use of less toxic swimming pool treatments are available, however, using more natural methods is not standard practice. One compromise is to request that the child limit time in the water, wear goggles, and wash off immediately after leaving the pool. Yet, others may not be able to tolerate the chemical exposure at all.

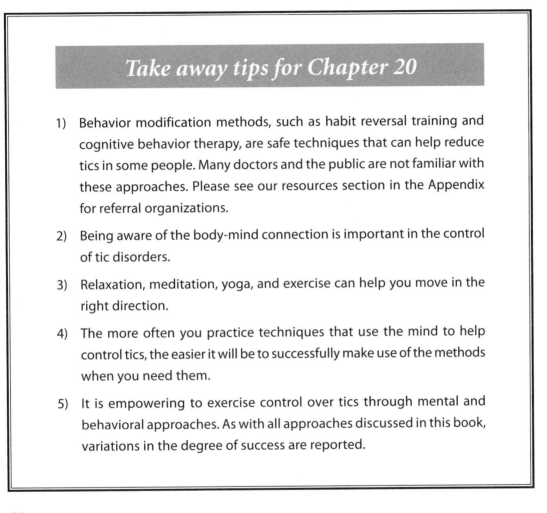

Take away tips for Chapter 20

1) Behavior modification methods, such as habit reversal training and cognitive behavior therapy, are safe techniques that can help reduce tics in some people. Many doctors and the public are not familiar with these approaches. Please see our resources section in the Appendix for referral organizations.

2) Being aware of the body-mind connection is important in the control of tic disorders.

3) Relaxation, meditation, yoga, and exercise can help you move in the right direction.

4) The more often you practice techniques that use the mind to help control tics, the easier it will be to successfully make use of the methods when you need them.

5) It is empowering to exercise control over tics through mental and behavioral approaches. As with all approaches discussed in this book, variations in the degree of success are reported.

Notes:

_____

_____

_____

_____

CHAPTER

21

Other Approaches

EEG biofeedback

ELECTROENCEPHALOGRAM (EEG) BIOFEEDBACK, also known as *neurofeedback,* has many applications and is an established treatment for reducing anxiety, pain, and hypertension. Recent studies have shown it is helpful for ADHD in 75% of those treated. It is also being used for conduct disorder, oppositional defiant disorder, learning problems and language processing, as well as irritable bowel syndrome, headache, seizures, and stroke conditions.

The general technique uses electronic equipment to relay information to participants about their brain's activity or to measure other body responses. The goal is to gain the ability to control the body to increase or decrease a specific response as shown on a monitor. It has been referred to as "exercising the brain." A skilled practitioner adjusts the approach for a particular condition, the part of the brain involved, and the types of symptoms a client is experiencing.

It is not unusual that 40 to 60 sessions of biofeedback are required to bring about long-lasting change in the disorders for which it is used. Equipment for home use is available for purchase, and some health insurance plans cover biofeedback intervention for select conditions.

To our knowledge, while there is no published research on biofeedback in the treatment of tics and TS, there may be a potential use of this treatment. Siegfried Othmer, PhD, chief scientist of EEG Spectrum International and co-author of the book *ADD: The 20-Hour Solution,* advised ACN:

Siegfried Othmer, PhD:

From the standpoint of neurofeedback, OCD and TS have a lot in common. They involve the same set of brain circuits, with symptom presentation just being somewhat different for both. One common element is over-arousal. In the vast majority of cases, the brain is overly engaged, restless, or even racing. There is a high degree of excitability of the motor system. The overarching need is for these brains to experience calming, both in general and specifically in regard to motor circuits.

> "Just as Ritalin can worsen tics, the standard neurofeedback approaches to ADHD can potentially worsen TS and OCD symptoms. A more specifically targeted approach is needed, so it is important to seek out an experienced clinician."
>
> —Siegfried Othmer, PhD

When such calming is achieved, both the tics (motor and vocal) and the OCD symptoms may be helped. What may someone expect from neurofeedback training for TS? First of all, this application of neurofeedback would be generally regarded as experimental. Also, most neurofeedback practitioners are oriented toward ADHD and may have little to no experience with TS and OCD. Just as Ritalin can worsen tics, the standard neurofeedback approaches to ADHD can potentially worsen TS and OCD symptoms. A more specifically targeted approach is needed, so it is important to seek out an experienced clinician. With the right approach, there should be significant improvement in symptoms in most cases. TS is a condition that appears to benefit from long-term training when the hoped-for symptom remediation is not quickly achieved. Such training can be done on a supervised home-training basis. The reader is referred to two recent books: *A Symphony in the Brain* by Jim Robbins, and *Getting Rid of Ritalin,* by Robert Hill, PhD, and Ed Castro, MD.

Homeopathy

Homeopathy is a system of healing designed to help the body balance itself. Discovered 200 years ago and practiced worldwide, its therapeutic action is still not fully understood. A point of contention for some conventional practitioners is the fact that therapeutic doses are so diluted, it seems impossible they could stimulate the body to correct its imbalances. Yet, not understanding why a treatment works is more common in the field of medicine than many realize. Research supports the use of homeopathy for numerous chronic and acute conditions.

Results of a survey by the Association for Comprehensive NeuroTherapy (ACN), published in the *Journal of Child and Adolescent Psychopharmacology* (2004) showed that homeopathy is one of the most popular alternative therapy methods pursued by those with tic disorders. Additional study is needed to determine the types of homeopathic treatment that are most useful, and to predict who is most likely to benefit.

Dana Ullman, MPH, an internationally recognized homeopath, explained how remedies are selected for a patient: "Professional homeopaths interview the client in detail to discover the totality of physical, emotional, and mental systems. They then refer to a toxicology text that outlines specific physical, emotional, and mental symptoms that various substances cause in overdose. Homeopaths seek to select the substance that would cause similar symptoms to those the person is experiencing. Highly diluted, specially prepared doses of that substance are then administered. Homeopathic remedies do not cause lasting side effects or addictions, and are therefore safe."

> "Homeopaths seek to select the substance that would cause similar symptoms to those the person is experiencing. Highly diluted, specially prepared doses of that substance are then administered. Homeopathic remedies do not cause lasting side effects or addictions, and are therefore safe."
>
> —Dana Ullman, MPH

Judith Reichenberg-Ullman, ND, LCSW, gives the following explanation in a new book (*A Drug-Free Approach to Asperger Syndrome and Autism*): "Natural substances are specially prepared as homeopathic medicine through a process of successive dilutions, and are given in small doses. For example, the homeopathic medicine *Apis* (most homeopathic medicines have Latin names) is derived from the honeybee. When a person suffers a bee sting, *Apis* will significantly reduce the pain, inflammation, and swelling. The reason for this is that these are the very symptoms that a bee sting causes in a healthy person."

The homeopathic remedy itself is usually in the form of a small pellet; tinctures, gels, powders and creams are also used. Sometimes a remedy can quickly resolve the problem. Other times, the treatment period can be lengthy, with several remedies used over time. Natural food stores carry a selection of homeopathic remedies. However, homeopaths suggest that for chronic conditions a professional should be consulted.

Amy Rothenberg, ND on treating tics with homeopathy

ACN consulted with Amy Rothenberg, a naturopathic doctor with special expertise in homeopathy, for information specific to treating tics with this approach. She and her husband Paul Herscu, ND, are directors of the New England School of Homeopathy, Amherst, Massachusetts. Dr. Rothenberg confirmed that TS can in some cases be successfully treated with homeopathy.

> We always treat the whole person with a constitutional homeopathic remedy based on the way he or she exhibits their particular problem, how that fits into overall health, physical symptoms (eg, do they usually feel warm/chilly, are there food cravings, what is the typical sleep position) and how that fits with his or her mental and emotional concerns.
>
> We do not treat Tourette syndrome (TS) per se, rather the person with TS. Paul and I have had good results with tic disorders and TS. For many, these symptoms are a sign that things are out of balance. We also try to help the patient understand what the stresses are in their lives that are pushing them over the brink toward symptoms.
>
> We work with patients over a lifetime. What we are looking for is that they move in a direction of health; we really do not work much with the concept of cure, because people evolve and their problems ebb and flow. There are no shortcuts, easy answers, or lists of common remedies. Some are born with healthier vital forces or have support systems and other therapies that work simultaneously to help with the process. Others are in a setting where it is more difficult for healing to occur. Sometimes a person improves to the point that he or she no longer considers themselves someone with TS, while others may

Detoxification

Detoxification is the process by which our bodies cleanse themselves of contaminants and toxins. It is normal for the body to maintain a state of balance and purity that is continually fostered by the body's functions and systems. We detoxify when we perspire, when we urinate or pass stools, and when we exhale. Drinking pure water, eating nutrient-rich foods, exercising, breathing fresh air, and avoiding contact with allergens facilitates the process.

However, our bodies were not designed to constantly detoxify the growing number of contaminants we currently encounter. An onslaught of industrialized products, food additives, and pesticides has resulted in multiple toxins accumulating in our bloodstreams and tissues, potentially harming numerous organs and systems in the body. The list includes harmful metals such as mercury, cadmium, aluminum, and lead, as well as a growing number of chemicals. A study in 2005 of a small sample of newborns revealed 287 chemicals were present in the umbilical cords, and over 200 of these had never been detected in cord blood previously. Many of these are toxic to the nervous system.

In an effort to rid the body of contaminants, health practitioners may recommend a range of detoxification treatments, such as nutrient and herbal "flushes," Epsom salt soaks, oral or intravenous chelation (for removal of toxic metals), oral or intravenous high dose antioxidants and glutathione, enemas, or saunas to help patients excrete toxins through the skin, urine, and colon. The use of these types of treatments should be evaluated carefully and monitored by a qualified professional.

Chelation therapy is being studied at the University of Arizona as an intervention for autism. Skilled, expert care is needed for chelation treatment; if pursued improperly it can have an adverse effect. Research on the use of detoxification methods specific to tic disorders is lacking. It is, however, a potential approach to consider if abnormally high levels of neurotoxins are identified and symptoms warrant this intervention. Current recommendations on detoxification methods are being explored by the Defeat Autism Now group, sponsored through the Autism Research Institute, San Diego (*www.autism.com/ari*). The Health Research Institute (outside Chicago) is studying nutritional approaches to assist in the detoxification process (*www.hriptc.org*). Look for updates on this important topic in our *Latitudes Online* issues.

now understand how to keep the disorder to a slight minimum. I have seen the spectrum—that is, one remedy was used and there were no more tics ever. For another person, I may need to work for years managing the symptoms.

Dr. Rothenberg pointed out that homeopathic medicines can be used along with conventional drug therapy, but the doses may need to be adjusted. The Resources section in the Appendix contains contact information for organizations that provide referral information for homeopathic practitioners.

Bodywork

Bodywork can be beneficial for tic disorders on two fronts. One is to determine whether a structural problem is causing or aggravating tics. A second benefit is being able to address muscle and nerve connections that have become stressed as a result of chronic ticcing. Bodywork is a broad area of practice, with only a few of the many approaches discussed here.

Osteopathic manipulative treatment and related approaches: Osteopathic physicians are trained in conventional or allopathic medicine as well as osteopathic manipulative treatment. Manipulation involves hands-on adjustments to the spine and other areas of the body to facilitate healing. Not all osteopathic physicians are skilled in this area beyond their initial training, nor do many currently incorporate these techniques into their practice.

Training at osteopathic medical schools promotes manipulation to address structural blockages or injuries that can result in abnormal circulation and changes in nerve impulses. The structural difficulties may have occurred at birth or be the result of accident, illness, poor posture, or stress. Overall body healing can be achieved more quickly and more completely when structural difficulties are corrected. Studies on osteopathic manipulative treatment have proven its effectiveness for a range of physical and psychologic problems. Physicians who specialize in osteopathic manipulative therapy can be located through the American Academy of Osteopathy, Indianapolis, Indiana (*www. academyofosteopathy.org*).

Cranial therapy, developed by William G. Sutherland, DO, is a form of osteopathic manipulation that provides a gentle hands-on treatment of the cranial bones of the skull and is practiced by some osteopathic physicians. These professionals can often be located through the Cranial Academy in Indianapolis, Indiana (*www.cranialacademy.org*).

John Upledger, DO, further developed this technique into a model that has grown in popularity and is used by tens of thousands of physicians, dentists, chiropractors, nurses, physical therapists, and other professional bodyworkers. He coined the term craniosacral therapy. This technique is taught worldwide through the Upledger Institute in Palm Beach Gardens, Florida (*www.upledger.com*).

ACN has received a few reports that osteopathic manipulative therapy, cranial osteopathy, and craniosacral therapy were helpful as part of a multidisciplinary approach to reducing tic symptoms. Studies have not yet been conducted on these applications to tics.

Chiropractic therapy: Doctors of Chiropractic traditionally treat illness and injuries with manipulation of the spinal column. Unlike osteopathic physicians, they do not have a medical degree. Chiropractors may focus on natural wellness approaches, such as physical therapy, nutrient therapy with supplements, diet, exercise, and lifestyle changes to aid in the body's healing process. Many practitioners have their own area of specialty, such as acupuncture.

> Chiropractors may focus on natural wellness approaches, such as physical therapy, nutrient therapy with supplements, diet, exercise, and lifestyle changes to aid in the body's healing process. Many practitioners have their own area of specialty, such as acupuncture.

Erin Elster, DC, certified by the International Upper Cervical Chiropractic Association, has documented the only published research on tics and bodywork. Dr. Elster told ACN: "A link between traumas to the head and/or neck (resulting in neck injuries) and the onset of Tourette syndrome has been established in medical literature. Possible traumas that can result in upper neck injuries include blows to the head, concussion, whiplash, falls, as well as automobile and sporting accidents. Often, traumatic births, such as those requiring the use of forceps or vacuum extraction, can also lead to upper neck injuries. These neck injuries can potentially lead to malfunctions within the brainstem and abnormal neurochemical levels, resulting in the onset of TS and other neurologic conditions."

Dr. Elster reported on successful treatment of a small number of TS cases through chiropractic care.

Massage: It is difficult to imagine the ongoing pain from repetitive muscle jerks that can occur thousands of times per day for some. Massage is a practical intervention to soothe tired muscles and increase relaxation. Massage can also reduce stress and enhance one's mood. In a study with children diagnosed as having ADHD, a twenty-minute massage twice a week for one month resulted in the children's mood being improved in the short-term, and classroom behavior improved for a longer period. Although we are unaware of research that investigates the effect of massage on tics, it may be similarly helpful.

Parents often feel helpless when it comes to reducing the physical pain of repeated tics. Yet, they can learn to offer a comforting massage. It may be best to experiment to learn what kind of touch—light or firm—feels best.

Energy medicine

A range of natural approaches fall under the category of *energy medicine*, a field in which practitioners use subtle energy fields to bring about physical and emotional change. Diverse examples include: hands-on treatments to remove energy blockages, variations on acupuncture and homeopathy, some types of yoga, Reiki, emotional freedom technique, somatoemotional release, Nambudripad's allergy elimination technique (NAET), healing from a distance, prayer, acupressure, muscle testing, and many others. Electrodermal testing devices have been developed with the goal of measuring subtle energy levels and providing readouts that direct therapeutic recommendations. These practices or techniques vary widely, and it is unfair to group them all together; we have only done so here in the interest of space. Research has barely started to bring some level of credibility to these efforts. While this lack of research does not reflect on their potential for healing, it does make it more difficult for the consumer to know where to turn.

ACN has received dramatic reports of tic reduction as a result of energy medicine treatment. However, the evidence is insufficient to recommend specific applications. Furthermore, some therapists may not have medical training and therefore could misjudge a situation, resulting in time lost in appropriate treatment when the patient actually had a physical condition that needed prompt standard or skilled integrative medical attention.

NAET is one of the fastest growing energy treatments. According to the founder, Devi S. Nambudripad, MD, the brain sends out a physical warning when there are blockages within the energy pathways of the body. These warnings can include inflammation, fever, and physiologic/psychologic disorders, among others. NAET aims to remove these harmful energy blockages. Practitioners report that NAET helps people regain health, which includes eliminating their allergies. We know that allergies or sensitivities to food and other substances may be associated with tics, and as such, NAET may be a treatment to consider on an experimental basis.

Some practitioners create spin-off approaches to NAET or other energy therapies that make finding such therapies more confusing for anyone considering their use. If you choose to explore any of these techniques, take the time to locate someone who has an excellent reputation. The therapist's experience in treating tics is not as much of a priority as are his or her integrity and skill. Also check whether certification is required in whatever field of therapy you are considering.

Chinese medicine

An intriguing study was published out of Beijing, China in 1996. Dr. L. Wu and colleagues at the First Affiliated Hospital, Tianjin College of Traditional Chinese Medicine, reported that acupuncture was "effective" in 92% of 156 children with TS. The "cure" rate was more than 70% and highest among children aged 11 to 15 years. These statistics are much higher than those achieved through any studied therapy for TS. ACN was naturally anxious to learn more about this research. (We had received a small number of reports on successful treatment of tics or TS with acupuncture.)

With the persistent help of Rick Ma, a Chinese-speaking *Latitudes* subscriber, ACN contacted Dr. Wu. He told Rick that we were the first from the West to ask him about his published study on TS. He explained that he believes a weakness in kidney essence, or insufficient "qi" (vital

> With the persistent help of Rick Ma, a Chinese-speaking *Latitudes* subscriber, ACN contacted the lead researcher, Dr. Wu. He told Rick that we were the first from the West to ask him about his published study on TS.

energy) is an underlying issue in Tourette's that exists from birth. He found that most of the children he worked with in the study under discussion overate or had improper diets, and he recognizes that stress increases symptoms. Dr. Wu attributes his success in treating older children to the fact that they were more willing than younger children to receive acupuncture treatments. The doctor indicated that he uses the same general acupuncture techniques as are used in the West but that the acupuncture points he uses may differ. He feels those who require only minimal or moderate amounts of medication before being treated are most likely to benefit.

On further investigation, we learned that the symptom profile required for a diagnosis of TS in this study was much more lax than is typical in the West. Other issues also arose that make the study results appear less robust. This is not to say that acupuncture does not hold promise, only that the high response rate for Dr. Wu's specific treatment may not be applicable to cases with more stringent criteria for a TS diagnosis.

ACN requested Dr. Robert Murdoch, a licensed acupuncture physician in Naples, Florida, to review Dr. Wu's research related to the treatment plan used. He replied: "The type of acupuncture used in Dr. Wu's study is *TCM acupuncture*, the traditional Chinese medicine hybrid system formulated by Mao Tse Tung. Traditional Chinese medicine includes acupuncture, diet, massage and manipulation, and herbology. It has a particular format for explaining disease patterns, distinct from other styles of medicine and other styles of acupuncture. There are many TCM practitioners in the United States, as it is the predominant style here. There are also many other approaches to acupuncture presently being used in the United States."

Without additional information and extended follow-up of the participants in Dr. Wu's study, Dr. Murdoch suggests that the research results, an important pioneering effort, need to be interpreted with caution.

A comprehensive review of Chinese medicine and TS: An excellent article in *The Journal of Chinese Medicine* (October 2003) reviews literature and case reports on Chinese medicine as a therapy for TS: "Tourette's Syndrome and Chinese Medicine: Treatment Possibilities" (in English) by Simon Becker. Becker summarizes the Chinese-language literature and provides insights on treating symptoms of TS based on his own training as well as the clinical experiences of other researchers and clinicians. He points out that TS is not frequently seen in Chinese medical practices and that it has not been widely discussed in medical journals. In fact, an equivalent to the term *Tourette syndrome* does not exist in traditional Chinese medical literature. This lack of terminology, Becker explains, does not mean the disorder is not treated; rather, the classification of symptoms differs.

In the reports Simon examined, some of the patients were said to have TS, yet when seeking treatment they had experienced symptoms for less than one month. Typically, a TS diagnosis requires that symptoms are present, at least intermittently, for one year.

Simon suggests that treating TS with Chinese medicine is "difficult." He concludes from his review of the research and contact with practitioners that for best results, the Chinese medical practice should be implemented as soon after tic symptoms occur as possible. Readers can contact *The Journal of Chinese Medicine,* available at: *www.jcm. co.uk* to purchase a copy of this article, which appears to be the most exhaustive report available on the use of acupuncture and other Chinese medicine approaches for TS.

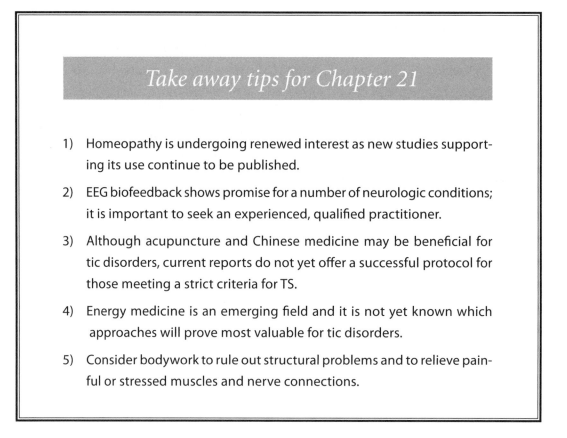

Take away tips for Chapter 21

1) Homeopathy is undergoing renewed interest as new studies supporting its use continue to be published.

2) EEG biofeedback shows promise for a number of neurologic conditions; it is important to seek an experienced, qualified practitioner.

3) Although acupuncture and Chinese medicine may be beneficial for tic disorders, current reports do not yet offer a successful protocol for those meeting a strict criteria for TS.

4) Energy medicine is an emerging field and it is not yet known which approaches will prove most valuable for tic disorders.

5) Consider bodywork to rule out structural problems and to relieve painful or stressed muscles and nerve connections.

Notes:

_____

_____

_____

_____

_____

SECTION EIGHT

Getting Started

CHAPTER

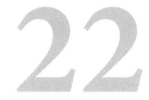

Finding Professional Help

A LIST OF ASSOCIATIONS FOR LICENSED or certified practitioners, from naturopathic doctors to behavioral specialists, is included in the resources section. Most of these organizations provide referral lists to help you in your search for help.

Many of the reports of positive treatment approaches received by ACN focus on diet, allergy, and nutritional supplements. The following forward-thinking physician organizations concentrate on these issues.

The American Academy of Environmental Medicine (AAEM)
www.aaem.com

The American Academy of Environmental Medicine is made up of osteopathic physicians and MDs who use specialized allergy testing methods, make recommendations for environmental adjustments, and develop nutritional therapies. A list of AAEM physician referrals is available on their website, with specialty areas noted for each. To be a "fellow" of the academy, one has to complete all course work and pass an examination. For "member" status, the requirements are less stringent, but the physicians will have attended some required courses in environmental medicine, in addition to their own medical specialty areas. Because these doctors are spread throughout the United

States and they are a relatively modest number to begin with, it may be difficult to find someone near you. (A small number of these practitioners can be found in some other countries.) Also, some include other approaches in their practices, so do not look for consistency throughout this organization (or the two groups that follow). Many of the positive responses you have read about in this book are the result of treatments provided by doctors in this group.

American College for Advancement in Medicine (ACAM)
www.acam.org

The American College for Advancement in Medicine's (ACAM's) primary focus is prevention and nutritional therapy. These practitioners have a wide range of medical backgrounds. This organization is one of the fastest growing and most established groups of integrative and alternative professionals in the country. Meetings are held regularly and are open to nonphysician healthcare professionals. Many doctors in ACAM specialize in nutrition, and chelation (removal of toxic metals from the body) or other therapies for detoxification. See the referral list on the ACAM website for members' specialty areas.

Defeat Autism Now (DAN)
www.autism.com/ari

These practitioners support the use of the Defeat Autism Now (DAN) medical protocol. This comprehensive approach, spearheaded by Bernard Rimland, PhD, has been developed by national leaders in the research and clinical fields and is updated at intervals. The protocols used have successfully reversed autism in some cases. Visit their website for a listing of healthcare practitioners. Some professionals on this list only see patients with autism; however, some of their protocols are also applicable to tic disorders. Be aware that the amount of training and experience in the use of the DAN protocol varies greatly within this list. If your physician is interested in the type of therapies included in this approach to correct biological imbalances, he or she should order: *Autism: Effective Biomedical Treatments* by Sidney Baker, MD and Jon Pangborn, PhD (available through *Amazon.com*).

✤

There are certainly excellent physicians and other types of practitioners offering integrative/alternative methods who do not belong to any of these groups, and everyone in the above organizations will not necessarily be helpful to you.

It is a matter of finding the right match for your situation. The search is often not easy, but it can be well worth the effort. As mentioned elsewhere in this book, financial considerations can be a significant barrier for many who seek comprehensive treatments when they do not have insurance, or when diagnostic methods and treatments are not covered by insurance. That said, many approaches described in this book can be undertaken with minimal financial expenditure.

Take away tips for Chapter 22

1) Your medical needs, location, and resources will all play a role in your search for professionals.

2) A multidisciplinary approach is often needed. Take advantage of the resources in the Appendix to locate practitioners.

3) The field of alternative and integrative medicine has made great strides over the last ten years, and major changes will continue to take place in this field.

4) You may need to educate professionals about your tic symptoms. They will not all be familiar with treating tic disorders, and will often be applying their expertise to your condition in a holistic manner.

Notes:

_____

_____

_____

_____

_____

_____

CHAPTER

Ten Tips for Success

TICS AND TOURETTE'S HAS PRESENTED A GREAT DEAL of information about the possible causes of tic symptoms and potential ways of dealing with them. Some of you are anxious to start investigating, immediately exploring which methods might work for you. Others may be in situations that require you to move more slowly. In both instances, it is helpful to organize your thoughts and develop a plan. This chapter will help you determine your next steps. Here are some pointers that others have found helpful in starting and maintaining their efforts.

1. Involve the whole family

Your chances for success are much greater when the immediate family joins the effort to have a healthier lifestyle. When someone is on a special diet, it is not easy to resist favorite treats when these items are stocked in the kitchen or are being openly enjoyed by others. There will be enough temptations to face outside the home!

Clean out your cupboards and refrigerator, and restock with nutritious foods. Reserve treats for special occasions, and try to select foods and beverages that are the least "harmful." For example, when there's a party, a small amount of ginger ale or natural beverage can usually be better tolerated than a large serving of artificially colored orange soda; natural potato chips will be well-tolerated compared with other chips that have added chemical flavors and colorings.

Ideally, all family members would understand the importance of eliminating triggers, whether it is a scented shampoo or dust in a bedroom. Request that grandparents or other relatives where your child frequently visits keep a "green" home—one without toxic chemicals or scented products. Inform relatives or friends who want to indulge the child with prohibited items that these are actually harmful to the youngster's health. Remember—we said "ideally." This request will be more successful with some than others.

2. Log your observations

Theron G. Randolph, MD, is credited with reporting the first medical case of chemical sensitivity more than 50 years ago. He was able to make this landmark discovery by keeping a running journal. Dr. Randolph was working with a woman who was plagued with asthma, fatigue, irritability, depression, and even loss of consciousness. All other doctors had given up on her case. Many assumed it was an emotional issue, but Dr. Randolph was determined to help her. Each time they met, he interviewed her at length about her symptoms and her daily life. Over a period of years, he recorded more than 40 pages of single-spaced notes.

One day, while reading through this record, Dr. Randolph had an "ah-ha" moment. It dawned on him that the patient's symptoms worsened when she was exposed to petrochemicals: burning coal, oil, gas, or their by-products. This reaction to chemicals was something that had not previously been considered in medicine. Once the cause had been identified, the woman was able to be successfully treated. With this one case, Dr. Randolph broke the mold of traditional medical evaluation and treatment, and he began teaching others how to look for environmental causes of symptoms. Had he not kept that log, he probably would never have made the connection.

A detailed log can help you identify triggers and will show you whether you are moving in the right direction. It only takes a few minutes to record your observations. Resist the temptation to stop keeping the log when things are going well, or when you are stumped. Perseverance will pay off!

3. Think outside the box

As you consider possible triggers for tics, don't be surprised if you become confused now and then. After all, based on ACN's survey results (Chapter 4), there are more than 50 types of possible triggers. You are not in a controlled laboratory setting where you can make observations while everything around you stays constant. While you are in the process of working on one trigger, another one (or two or three!) may rise to the surface.

Here is an example: Let's say a mother worked hard to change her daughter's diet to focus on low-sugar, high-nutrient foods. She also made changes at home to reduce chemical exposures, dust, and other allergens. She saw some improvement in symptoms and was starting to feel encouraged when one day her daughter—let's call her Sonia—came home with a major flare-up in tics after spending the day at a new friend's home.

Sonia is aware that her tics have increased and insists she has no idea what could be responsible; she says she avoided foods she reacts to and nothing out of the ordinary occurred. The mom asks questions about the friend's home but, with no obvious answers emerging, she starts to feel frustrated.

This mother needs to recognize that she can't, at that moment, possibly know everything that might have triggered the reaction. Perhaps the friend's home was sprayed with pesticides the previous day and that exposure is causing the response. The family might own a dog, and a possible dog allergy has never been considered. Sonia may not be telling the truth about what was eaten. Possibly the home contains scented plug-ins or was recently cleaned with strong chemical cleansers. Maybe the new friend teased Sonia about her tics, and this raised the daughter's stress level, resulting in more tics. Or, Sonia could be coming down with an infection that is affecting the immune system. The list goes on . . . .

The point is, don't be discouraged when causes or triggers are not obvious. Just document what happens. Explore possible triggers when you can, and watch for a pattern to emerge as time goes on.

We've included an example of creative problem-solving on the next page. This list presents numerous issues that might be involved when tics increase while in a car. Try not to be overwhelmed by all the potential "players" in a given situation. Instead, look at

Creative Problem Solving

This is an example of a complex trigger situation: A son complains to his parents that his tics are worse when he is in the family car. Why might this happen? Let's think it through by reviewing the possibilities:

1) Does this occur only when the vehicle is moving (motion-related), or does the reaction begin whenever he is seated in the car?

2) Does the problem occur only with this particular car or when riding in other vehicles as well?

3) Are chemicals involved? Does the car have a new-car smell, stain-treated upholstery, scented air-freshener, smoke odors, or a faulty exhaust system?

4) Are the textures or the feeling of the seat fabric irritating or distressing to him?

5) Is there anxiety associated with being among other passengers, being in an enclosed space, or with the destination (ie, doesn't want to go to school)?

6) Does it only occur after school or with some other event during which he was making an effort to withhold tics and is now letting them out?

7) Is the carpet or upholstery moldy or musty?

8) Is the temperature in the car a problem—is there an adequate heater or air conditioner?

9) Is the response a reaction to visual stimuli? Are the tics worse when scenery is rapidly moving past? Are there complaints that the sunlight is too bright?

10) Is the response worse when on crowded freeways where there is a higher concentration of exhaust? Is noise level a factor?

You can record your ideas for complex situations on the Brainstorming Tic Triggers worksheet, page 101; plan to review the worksheet when you have additional insights.

them as opportunities to investigate, when time allows. As you gain experience in tracking down triggers, it will be easier for you to unravel the issues involved.

It is no exaggeration to say that you have to be a detective! You must decide for yourself how vigorously you want to explore the leads you find. Although it may not be feasible to track down all of them, if you remain alert and open to possibilities, you will be able to get to the bottom of situations more easily.

4. Use a comprehensive approach

One of the biggest mistakes people make when trying to use natural methods is to focus on just one or two areas, missing the big picture. They might concentrate on nutritional supplements and ignore chemicals in the environment. Or, they might initiate a natural diet and ignore dust and mold allergies. When your efforts are too limited, your results will be disappointing. It's best to gradually expand your circle of focus to be as comprehensive as needed to reduce symptoms.

> When your efforts are too limited, your results will be disappointing. It's best to gradually expand your circle of focus to be as comprehensive as needed to reduce symptoms.

With this in mind, you may need to consult different types of practitioners when you are dealing with a difficult case, and ask them to collaborate when appropriate.

5. Avoid being rigid

There are no easy answers when it comes to finding the right treatments for tics, whether using conventional or alternative methods. Some people use medications for tics and related conditions and report good results. If you need to use conventional drugs, don't feel guilty about it. Take heart that alternative approaches can often reduce the amount of medication needed. It is possible to benefit from both conventional and complementary medicine.

The Association for Comprehensive NeuroTherapy never gives specific advice about whether someone should take prescribed medications. As a general policy, we recommend that commonsense, natural approaches be followed whenever feasible, with medications used only when necessary. Yet, symptoms can be so serious that the physician and family decide medication is needed without waiting to try other methods. Sometimes, use of a medication can make a situation more manageable, allowing for natural treatments to be used. There are no hard and fast rules.

Some people embrace a holistic approach, yet are so dogmatic and purist in their efforts that they foster more resentment in the family than improvement in symptoms. Being too rigid and demanding in your outlook can backfire. Difficult decisions will need to be made, and flexibility along with a firm (not unyielding) resolve can help.

6. Accentuate the positive!

Give your child (or spouse, etc.) lots of hugs and encouragement, with sincere praise. Do you focus more on what went wrong than what went right? If so, you have lots of company—this is the norm, and it's not an easy habit to break. It has been said that it takes five positive comments to overcome the damage of one critical remark. Whether this is accurate or not, give it a try. Make your compliments or positive statements real—don't exaggerate.

Develop an awareness of how you communicate, and adjust your pattern, if needed. This will help ensure that those you care about are receiving adequate support and appreciation with a minimum of negativity, and this in itself will reduce stress. It's also a good idea to show appreciation for efforts made by everyone involved in this quest for health. Don't take their cooperation for granted.

7. Share the message

Once you find something is helpful, such as diet or a clean, nontoxic environment, share this information with relatives, friends, co-workers, school officials, and others. Not only will this help educate them, but it will also encourage them to make the changes necessary to accommodate you or your child. It is not unheard of for an office building to be declared a no-perfume zone, or for employees to bring air filters to work. Parents can request pesticide spray schedules at schools and encourage natural pest management.

Take time to speak with teachers about food in the classroom, at lunch, and in after-school programming, and ask for their cooperation. You will not be the first parent to do so. No one has the right to feed your child foods or beverages that are harmful.

Addressing food issues at school without making the student feel singled out or deprived takes tactful communication, but it can be done. There are some schools that do not allow junk foods in the classroom or on campus. This is a growing trend, but not yet practiced in most schools. You can play an important role in initiating change.

> No one has the right to feed your child foods or beverages that are harmful. Addressing food issues at school without making the student feel singled out or deprived takes tactful communication, but it can be done.

You are your child's advocate. Once your child is old enough to discuss the topic, find out how he or she feels about you talking to others about tics or other symptoms. Some children are remarkably resilient and upfront about their condition while others feel terribly self-conscious. Keep their wishes in mind when talking with teachers, friends, or relatives. This doesn't mean that you don't tell anyone if the child requests this, but honor the wish as much as is feasible by using care in the way you speak and by requesting confidentiality on the part of the listener.

Leslie E. Parker, PhD, has quality, reader-friendly material on TS and PANDAS on her website (see *www.tourettesyndrome.net*). Many of these articles are helpful for sharing with educators. The national Tourette Syndrome Association (*www.tsa-usa.org*) also has conventional material on how tic disorders can affect the school experience, with ideas for teachers and parent advocacy; material by Susan Conners is excellent.

When you learn that something in the school environment is aggravating your child's tics or is a potential health concern, such as mold or the use of toxic cleaning products or scented air fresheners, talk to the school staff and share your expectations for the situation to improve. School officials often understand and respond when you speak of the problem in terms of allergies or hypersensitivities.

8. Recognize the value of self-discovery

As a child or adult begins to adapt to dietary changes or other adjustments in routine, some cheating is to be expected. Think of it as testing the waters. Be understanding and encourage an open dialogue about it, while trying to show that these actions have consequences. If you punish or scold every time there is a slip, it is less likely that you will be told about future lapses, making your efforts more frustrating. If you are the person with tics, use the same principle. Recognize that you will at times give in to temptation or relax your efforts—it's human nature. Just try to get back on track quickly.

It is to everyone's advantage to develop a reasonable amount of discipline. Using behavioral charts can help, especially for children who like to see their efforts documented and rewarded (see: *www.freebehaviorcharts.com*). Stick to regular sleep schedules and ensure adequate rest. As the immune system is strengthened, occasional lapses will be better tolerated.

Read next how a mother writing to ACN handled an incident with her eight-year-old child, after a setback in their previously successful plan:

> When Danny came home from school yesterday, he was verbally abusive to the family. I suspected from past experience that this was a reaction to something he had eaten—it is not his nature. (A year before, after much trial and error, we discovered which foods set off behavior and tic problems. These were chemical additives, sugars, and certain foods. By avoiding those, his tics and angry behavior disappeared. When he goes off his diet, I've noticed that behavior is the first thing affected.) I immediately asked what off-limits food he had eaten at school, but he denied eating anything he should not have had.
>
> The following day, when Danny had calmed down, I had a good talk with him about his actions and how food affects him. I tried to make him understand that the restrictive diet is not a punishment, and that he needs to follow it to help himself. We talked about the difference in his mood compared with his mood the previous day, and how those around him react to both types of behavior. He acknowledged that he understood why we were worried about his diet. Then Danny admitted that while at school the day before, he had eaten three candy bars given to him by schoolmates—items he had been unable to tolerate in the past. I felt he learned his lesson without me having to lecture him.

9. Follow your plan

Once you develop your intervention plans, stick with the interventions you decided on for six to eight weeks, or as directed by your practitioner. Try not to jump from one concept to another. It takes time for natural healing to occur. The more often you switch gears, the harder it will be to know what is working. ACN often hears reports such as, "I stopped caffeine for a week and didn't notice a difference, so I started drinking coffee again. I also tried some vitamins for a few weeks and they didn't seem to help."

It is not unusual to need to "fine-tune" treatment, so it is important to keep in close contact with your practitioner so results can be monitored and therapies adjusted, added or dropped. Don't give up at the first sign of frustration or lack of anticipated progress.

10. Take care of yourself

If you are dealing with a difficult case, reach out for the support you need to help you cope, through local support groups, friends and family, counseling, and reputable online forums. If you feel exceptionally stressed, anxious, or depressed, seek professional help.

Many parental "investigators" work full-time jobs and are pressed for time. Some have more than one child at home, and many have financial or other challenges. It is no small feat to juggle all the demands required to embark on a new path to health. If you start to feel pressured or exhausted from the special efforts you are making, take a break and coast for a while.

This is not a race, and you need to pace your efforts. You have to maintain a personal balance for the sake of all concerned. You may also realize that your child or others involved need a short break, too. Set aside some time for fun family activities where your concerns about healing are put on the back burner, and when no one focuses on symptoms.

Do not ignore your own body and self. When you give your child or other family members healthful food and nutritional supplements, don't forget your own nutritional needs. Remember to take time to exercise. And, carve out some time to allow quiet moments for spiritual renewal in whatever form is comfortable for you. Have hope, and be open to new possibilities of healing.

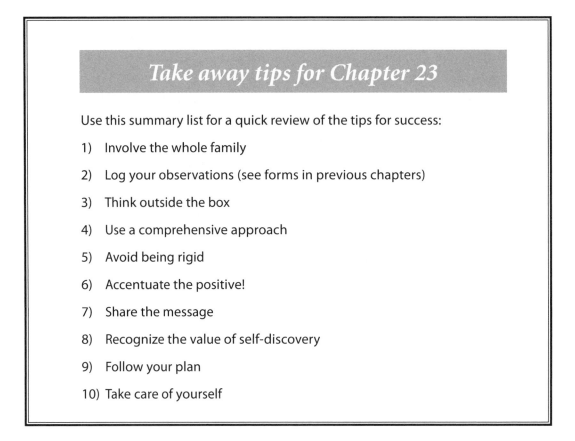

Take away tips for Chapter 23

Use this summary list for a quick review of the tips for success:

1) Involve the whole family

2) Log your observations (see forms in previous chapters)

3) Think outside the box

4) Use a comprehensive approach

5) Avoid being rigid

6) Accentuate the positive!

7) Share the message

8) Recognize the value of self-discovery

9) Follow your plan

10) Take care of yourself

Notes:

_____

_____

_____

_____

_____

_____

Afterword:
Moving Ahead
A note from the author

⁓

AFTER MANY YEARS OF WORKING TO DEVELOP and share this message, it is satisfying to know that through this book information on natural treatments for tics is finally available to a wide audience. However, my satisfaction is tempered by an awareness of the huge task that lies ahead.

Those reading this book, and the thousands who visit our website each day, will learn that diet, nutritional imbalances, allergens, the immune system, and chemicals in the environment can impact tics. They will also learn that a number of integrative and complementary therapies may help. Unfortunately, this leaves millions of others worldwide who are affected by tics and do not know that options exist, beyond drugs.

We have been sharing our findings with key leaders in the conventional field for 15 years. Still, the "standard line" on tics remains unchanged. To this day, strong tic medications continue to be prescribed to children as young as four years of age, with no discussion of natural approaches or even commonsense preventive efforts. Physicians who do present alternatives are the exception.

Why don't doctors consider these possibilities? They have been discouraged from doing so. Here is one of many such examples: In August 2004, an article written by a member of the Tourette Syndrome Association Medical Advisory Board was published in *Contemporary Pediatrics* and posted on the Tourette Syndrome Association's website.

In a bold, highlighted section, the misleading article said (excerpt):

KEY POINTS
Dispelling misconceptions about the
management of Tourette syndrome

FALLACY: Dietary modification, allergy testing, and environmental allergen control can minimize tics.

FACT: Despite the popular appeal of these approaches, any role they might have in the management of tics has yet to be proved.

Through this article, pediatricians were told that these natural methods of approaching tics are useless. The piece was subsequently summarized in the *New York Times* (January 2005). Not surprisingly, the author assumed the above statement was accurate and her column on Tourette syndrome concluded with a "caution" against "a common tendency for families to use a variety of alternative remedies and dietary restrictions, since none have proved useful." As a result, beyond the damage of the original article, more than a million additional readers received this unfortunate message.

Conventional medical groups often imply studies with natural treatments have had negative results—when the needed studies have not even been attempted.

Internet forums lit up with protests to the articles, but the damage had already been done. Why are people being discouraged from exploring something as basic and logical as dietary change or environmental adjustments to avoid allergic reactions when the traditional option is toxic drugs that have not even been tested for long-term use with children? (Yes, there are studies with adults for these strong drugs. The outcomes are unsatisfactory and the adverse effects worrisome. The mere existence of studies, per se, in no way implies a quality treatment.)

ACN has never claimed to have the answer for everyone, but everyone has a right to decide for themselves how they wish to approach tic disorders. They should be given complete and truthful information with which to do so.

Keeping our focus on the children

When I measure progress in this field, I often think of it in terms of childhood. Boys and girls who were seven years old when our movement started are now 22. We've helped some of these children, while most were offered nothing but drugs by their doctors, and parents were told not to waste their time looking for other answers. Many of these kids lost the chance for a normal childhood. Meanwhile, relevant research barely progressed.

What about those who are seven years old now? Can we reach them in time? I believe we can, by sponsoring our own research efforts. Further, we can build a team of professionals with multidisciplinary backgrounds who will collaborate and define the best ways to approach tics. Patients and families can network together, allowing our movement to grow at a faster pace. We can also hold conferences and take the message directly to the public.

We may not have drug companies lining our pockets, but that does not mean we are collectively without resources, nor should we ever be without a vision.

Let's help today's children—now.

ACN has four critical needs as we seek to increase the scientific understanding of tics and Tourette's and provide this message to others:

- *Physicians, practitioners, and researchers:* All who are willing to collaborate and share relevant findings and/or theories through a "think tank" process are urged to contact ACN as we aim to develop a comprehensive protocol for the treatment of tic disorders. Please sign up at *www.Latitudes.org* and we will be in touch with you.

- *Funding:* We need to dramatically increase resources for our research fund and to support ACN operations. (Please see our contact information on page 273 to participate in fundraising efforts, or to donate.)

- *Families and patients:* We encourage you to share your experiences with us as you explore natural treatments for tics. You can send your information by regular mail or through the *www.Latitudes.org* website. Communication is confidential, but please include your contact details for verification and follow-up.

- ***Volunteers:*** If you can assist with publicity, grant writing, marketing, networking or conference planning, please contact us through the Volunteer area on the *Latitudes.org* website.

Children everywhere are counting on us. If not us—then who? Now is the time to make a difference. Please see what you can do to help.

Thank you—Sheila J. Rogers

To Donate or Contact ACN

The Association for Comprehensive NeuroTherapy is a 501(c)3 nonprofit organization; all donations are fully tax-deductible.

Contributions are very much needed to expand our efforts and develop new research. Donations can be made online at our site www.Latitudes.org or sent by mail with a check payable to ACN. All donations will be gratefully acknowledged.

Association for Comprehensive NeuroTherapy
PO Box 2198, Broken Arrow, OK 74013

acn@Latitudes.org

Please see the following page for information on publications by ACN.

Publications by ACN

www.Latitudes.org

This is our main home website. "Latitudes" was selected for its meaning: "freedom of action or choice." Our site features cutting-edge material on natural approaches to depression, autism, anxiety, attention deficit disorders/hyperactivity, obsessive-compulsive disorder, Tourette's and tic disorders, and learning problems. *The following helpful publications are linked on our home page:*

Latitudes Online

This is the global web upgrade of our popular subscription-based magazine, *Latitudes* (the previous six volumes were in print format). *Latitudes Online* highlights articles by international experts, interviews, research updates, environmental tips, success stories, book reviews, and more. A subscription to *Latitudes Online* is the best way to stay updated on the latest findings for treating tics. We encourage you to take advantage of the convenient web access and subscribe now!

Better Brains, Naturally

This free online blog by Sheila J. Rogers can be read directly at *www.Latitudes.blogs.com*. If you aren't familiar with blogs, just go to the site and see how reader-friendly it is. Those who register for membership receive notices whenever Sheila posts a new message.

ACN Today

You will want to sign up for our organization's free electronic newsletter, *ACN Today*, to receive timely articles on health issues and updates on all of ACN's news—delivered right to your e-mail box.

ACN Forum

You can benefit from insights of others around the world by searching and accessing thousands of posted comments and suggestions on our forum. You can also post your own messages and questions. Just click on the forum link on our home page to get started.

Research & Resource Updates

Research Updates

New Recognition that Foods Affect ADHD

The American Academy of Pediatrics (AAP) made a landmark admission in February 2008 following publication of a new study on diet and attention deficit disorder/hyperactivity (ADHD):

"The overall findings of the study are clear and require that even we skeptics, who have long doubted parental claims of the effects of various foods on the behavior of their children, admit we might have been wrong.

—*AAP Grand Rounds,* a publication of the American Academy of Pediatrics

Here's a summary of the study under discussion, published in the *Lancet*:

A team of researchers at the University of Southampton in England conducted a double-blind study with 3-year-olds and 8- to 9-year-olds. Children were given either a test drink with additives, or a placebo, using additive levels typically consumed by British children. Behavior was rated by teachers, parents, and independent observers. The authors concluded that the results "lend strong support for the case that food additives exacerbate hyperactive behaviors (inattention, impulsivity, and overactivity) in children at least up to middle childhood."

McCann D., Barrett A., et al: "Food additives and hyperactive behaviour in 3-year-old and 8/9-year-old children in the community: a randomised, double-blinded, placebo-controlled trial"; *The Lancet* November 2007

Not long after the American Academy of Pediatrics admitted they might have been wrong by refusing to acknowledge reports of foods causing an increase in ADHD symptoms, the importance of the role of diet in ADHD was further supported by an editorial in the *British Journal of Medicine* by Andrew Kemp, MD, professor of pediatric allergy and immunology at the University of Sydney, Australia. Dr. Kemp recommended dietary intervention as "standard treatment" for children with attention deficit disorders.

The artificial colorings and preservatives used in the *Lancet* study are often included in cereals, snacks, vitamins, prescription drugs, and other processed items—not just candy. Several organizations have now called for a ban on artificial additives. Michael Jacobson, PhD, executive director of the Center for Science in the Public Interest, recommended in a letter to the *British Medical Journal*:

> Considering the numerous studies conducted over the past 30 years, Andrew Kemp is right in urging physicians to routinely encourage patients with hyperactivity to avoid food dyes. However, considering the dyes' lack of health benefit and the risk they pose, the proper public health approach is for national governments to ban the use of all food dyes. After all, it is extremely difficult, first, for a parent to determine that a child is sensitive to dyes and, second, for parents to protect easily tempted children from tasty colorful foods that are served at parties; sold at stores, restaurants, and vending machines; and traded among friends.

Jacobson points out that the British Food Standards Agency encouraged manufacturers and restaurants to switch to safer, natural colorings. As a result of government pressure, companies such as Kellogg, McDonalds, Kraft, and Mars now market foods without dyes in Britain, but market the same foods with dyes in the United States. He adds that the U.S. Food and Drug Administration maintains that "well-controlled studies conducted . . . have produced no evidence that food additives cause hyperactivity or learning disabilities in children."

In addition to the above study, research released in April of this year examined an elimination diet that resulted in improved ADHD symptoms; citation below.

Pelsser L., Frankena K., et al: "A randomized controlled trial into the effects of food on ADHD" *Eur Child Adolesc Psychiatry* published online April 2008.

The Influence of Food and Drink on Tics in Tourette Syndrome: A Misleading Study

Studies on diet and tics are severely lacking (see page 174 of this book). The only related study completed since the first edition of *Tics and Tourette's* is described in this article. German research published in April 2008 was designed to determine if food and drink affected tic symptoms of Tourette syndrome (TS). Unfortunately, limitations of the survey approach and a biased interpretation by the researchers resulted in misleading conclusions, perpetuating the false concept that food does not affect tics.

The study: A standardized questionnaire was sent to almost 900 people with TS. Respondents were asked to reply whether 32 different food products and substances influenced tics. The survey related to numerous motor and vocal tics; the products were: pork, beef, poultry, fish, dairy products, eggs, food containing yeast, wheat, rye, barley, oat and spelt, preserving agents, citrus fruits, juices, tomatoes, paprika, strongly seasoned food, potatoes, rice, refined white sugar, sweeteners, honey, chocolate, coke, coffee, black tea, beer, other alcoholic drinks, cigarettes, and marijuana, among others. Respondents were asked to indicate if they noticed an increase in tics after consuming any of these products. Forty percent filled the survey on behalf of their children.

About one-fourth of the group returned surveys. A significant number responded that an increase in tics was seen following consumption of coke, coffee, black tea, preserving agents, refined white sugar, and other sweeteners.

Further, restricted ("oligo-antigen") diets as well as a sugar-free diet were reported to result in improvements in symptoms.

Researchers' interpretation: The authors had hypothesized that food would not affect tics. Yet, based on survey results they acknowledged that caffeine indeed can worsen symptoms. As to the significant finding that preservatives and refined white sugar were also shown to increase tics, the authors dismissed this data. They suggested that the "stress" from guilt over eating junk food might have been what made the tics worse. Or, they say, perhaps people simply made the connection because they had heard these foods might affect ADHD. In other words, the researchers decided that respondents could be believed for their observations on caffeine—but other observations they made connecting food to tic symptoms were somehow not reliable. See this excerpt from the journal article:

> Respondents assessed a deterioration of tics after the consumption of preserving agents and white sugar. An interpretation of these results is . . . difficult. On the one hand, it has to be taken into consideration that it is general knowledge that the consumption of preserving agents and white sugar to excess is unhealthy. The consumption of these foods, therefore, might gnaw at one's conscience, thus might cause stress and this, in turn, might deteriorate [worsen] tics. On the other hand, afore mentioned foods are suspected to worsen several other disorders including ADHD, and therefore, people may tend to generalize the negative attribute of these foods.

Further, the authors of the study give little attention to the fact that restricted diets were seen to *improve* tic symptoms.

Further commentary from Sheila Rogers: One of the biggest drawbacks to a survey such as this is that people are not readily aware of potential tic responses to foods prior to completing the survey. Physicians do not encourage families to look for food reactions; in fact they often discourage it. Even the researchers for this study hypothesized that there would not be a connection between food, drink, and tics.

Except for obvious situations such as an immediate increase in tics after coffee consumption, it is often difficult to sort out tic reactions to common foods (like tomatoes, potatoes, dairy, and wheat). These foods are often eaten together at the same meal or throughout the same day. Further, not all food reactions are immediate, which complicates the picture.

Determining food sensitivities requires significant effort, as indicated in Sections 2 and 5 of this book. Keeping a food diary and using food elimination trials are two of the best methods; assistance from an experienced practitioner is often required, especially when tics are chronic.

In this study, it can be assumed that respondents gave their impressions without prior examination of specific food reactions, thereby overlooking possible connections to tic symptoms. In addition, 40% of respondents were parents speaking on behalf of their children. Children are even less aware of reactions and less able to express a connection between foods and tics. Further, parents are not always with their children in order to be aware of foods consumed and reactions.

When the survey shortcomings are combined with the researchers' off-handed dismissal of reports that certain foods aggravated tics and their further lack of attention to reports that restricted diets improved symptoms, it must be concluded that the published report does more harm than good.

> Müller-Vahl K.R., Buddensiek N., et al "The influence of different food and drink on tics in Tourette syndrome" *Acta Paediatr* 2008 Apr; 97(4):442–6.

Increased Rate of Tics Connected to Thimerosal in Vaccines

**Thimerosal exposure in infants and neurodevelopmental disorders:
An assessment of computerized medical records in the Vaccine Safety Datalink**

A study of mercury exposure from Thimerosal-containing vaccines administered from birth to 7 months and from birth to 13 months showed that increased mercury exposure increased the rate ratio for autism and autism spectrum disorders, attention deficit disorders, developmental and learning disorders, disturbance of emotions specific to childhood and adolescence, and tics.

The authors state: "For example, in the birth to 7 month period, the rate of tics was approximately 3.4 times higher given a 100 microgram increase in mercury exposure in Thimerosal-containing vaccines."

> Young H., et al: Thimerosal exposure in infants and neurodevelopmental disorders: An assessment of computerized medical records in the Vaccine Safety Datalink. J Neurol Sci 2008; 2008.04.002.

New Documentation on the Dangers of Scented Products

Reports to ACN indicate that scented items can aggravate tics and hyperactivity, and other neurological reactions are often experienced by some people. Environmental physicians routinely advise that scented personal and home products should be avoided. Their recommendation gained support from the study below. Sharing this article can help convince friends, family members, and schools to go unscented for the health benefit of all.

Toxic chemicals found in common scented laundry products, air fresheners
A press release from the University of Washington, July 23, 2008

A University of Washington (UW) study of top-selling laundry products and air fresheners found the products emitted dozens of different chemicals. All six products tested gave off at least one chemical regulated as toxic or hazardous under federal laws, but none of those chemicals was listed on the product labels.

"I first got interested in this topic because people were telling me that the air fresheners in public restrooms and the scent from laundry products vented outdoors were making them sick," said Anne Steinemann, a UW professor of civil and environmental engineering and public affairs. "And I wanted to know, 'What's in these products that is causing these effects?' " She analyzed the products to discover the chemicals' identity.

"I was surprised by both the number and the potential toxicity of the chemicals that were found," Steinemann said. Chemicals included acetone, the active ingredient in paint thinner and nail-polish remover; limonene, a molecule with a citrus scent; as well as acetaldehyde, chloromethane, and 1,4-dioxane.

"Nearly 100 volatile organic compounds were emitted from these six products, and none were listed on any product label. Plus, five of the six products emitted one or more carcinogenic 'hazardous air pollutants,' which are considered by the Environmental

Protection Agency to have no safe exposure level," Steinemann said.

Her study was published online by the journal *Environmental Impact Assessment Review.* Steinemann chose not to disclose the brand names of the six products she tested. In a larger study of 25 cleaners, personal care products, air fresheners and laundry products, now submitted for publication, she found that many other brands contained similar chemicals.

Because manufacturers of consumer products are not required to disclose the ingredients, Steinemann studied the products to discover their contents. She studied three common air fresheners (a solid deodorizer disk, a liquid spray, and a plug-in oil) and three laundry products (a dryer sheet, fabric softener, and a detergent), selecting a top seller in each category. She bought household items at a grocery store and asked companies for samples of industrial products.

In the laboratory, each product was placed in an isolated space at room temperature and the surrounding air was analyzed for volatile organic compounds, small molecules that evaporate from the product's surface into the air.

Results showed 58 different volatile organic compounds above a concentration of 300 micrograms per cubic meter, many of which were present in more than one of the six products. For instance, a plug-in air freshener contained more than 20 different volatile organic compounds. Of these, seven are regulated as toxic or hazardous under federal laws. The product label lists no ingredients, and information on the Material Safety Data Sheet, required for workplace handling of chemicals, lists the contents as "mixture of perfume oils."

This study does not address links between exposure to chemicals and health effects. However, two national surveys published by Steinemann and a colleague in 2004 and 2005 found that about 20% of the population reported adverse health effects from air fresheners, and about 10% complained of adverse effects from laundry products vented to the outdoors. Among asthmatics such complaints were roughly twice as common.

Manufacturers are not required to list the ingredients used in laundry products and air fresheners. Personal-care products and cleaners often contain similar fragrance chemicals, Steinemann said. And although cosmetics are required by the Food and Drug Administration to list ingredients, no law requires products of any kind to list chemicals used in fragrances.

"Fragrance chemicals are of particular interest because of the potential for involuntary exposure, or second-hand scents," Steinemann said.

"Be careful if you buy products with fragrance, because you really don't know what's in them," she added. "I'd like to see better labeling. In the meantime, I'd recommend that instead of air fresheners people use ventilation, and with laundry products, choose fragrance-free versions."

The European Union recently enacted legislation requiring products to list 26 fragrance chemicals when they are present above a certain concentration in cosmetic products and detergents. No similar laws exist in the United States.

"I hope this study will raise public awareness, and reduce exposures to potentially hazardous chemicals," said Steinemann.

For more information, contact Steinemann at (206) 616-2661 or acstein@u.washington.edu.

The Case for Precaution in the Use of Cell Phones

ACN has identified cell phone use as potential trigger for tics. Research suggests that there can be harmful neurological effects from cell phone radiation. The University of Pittsburgh Cancer Institute conducted a review of relevant studies and issued the following warning with recommendations (*July 2008 press release; edited for space*).

Advice from University of Pittsburgh Cancer Institute

Based on advice from an international expert panel, University of Pittsburgh Cancer Institute

Analysis of Recent Studies

Electromagnetic fields generated by cell phones should be considered a potential human health risk. Sufficient time has not elapsed in order for us to have conclusive data on the biological effects of cell phones and other cordless phones—a technology that is now universal.

Studies in humans do not indicate that cell phones are safe, nor do they yet clearly show that they are dangerous. But, growing evidence indicates that we should reduce exposures, while research continues on this important question.

Manufacturers report that cell and wireless phones emit electromagnetic radiation. Electromagnetic fields are likely to penetrate the brain of children more deeply than adults. The most recent studies, which include subjects with a history of cell phone usage for a duration of at least 10 years, show a possible association between certain benign tumors (acoustic neuromas) and some brain cancers on the side the device is used.

However, human epidemiological studies on cell phones conducted to date cannot be conclusive. Due to their recently increased use, we are not yet able to evaluate their long term impact on health. Even where an association between exposure and cancer is well established and the risk very high—as with tobacco and lung cancer—

under similar study conditions (in other words with people who smoked for less than 10 years) it would be difficult, if not impossible, to identify an increased risk of cancer, as the risk appears mostly 15 to 35 years later.

The Ten Precautions

Given the absence of definitive proof in humans of the carcinogenic effects of electromagnetic fields of cell phones, we cannot speak about the necessity of preventative measures (as for tobacco or asbestos). In anticipation of more definitive data covering prolonged periods of observation, the existing data press us to share important prudent and simple measures of precaution for cell phone users, as have been variously suggested by several national and international reports.

These measures are also likely to be important for people who are already suffering from cancer and who must avoid any external influence that may contribute to disease progression.

Practical advice to limit exposure to electromagnetic radiation emitted from cell phones:

1. Do not allow children to use a cell phone, except for emergencies. The developing organs of a fetus or child are the most likely to be sensitive to any possible effects of exposure to electromagnetic fields.

2. While communicating using your cell phone, try to keep the cell phone away from the body as much as possible. The amplitude of the electromagnetic field is one-fourth the strength at a distance of two inches and fifty times lower at three feet. Whenever possible, use the speaker-phone mode or a wireless Bluetooth headset, which has less than 1/100th of the electromagnetic emission of a normal cell phone. Use of a hands-free ear piece attachment may also reduce exposures.

3. Avoid using your cell phone in places like a bus, where you can passively expose others to your phone's electromagnetic fields.

4. Avoid carrying your cell phone on your body at all times. Do not keep it near your body at night such as under the pillow or on a bedside table, particularly if pregnant. You can also put it on "flight" or "off-line" mode, which stops electromagnetic emissions.

5. If you must carry your cell phone on you, make sure that the keypad is positioned toward your body and the back is positioned toward the outside so that the transmitted electromagnetic fields move away from your rather than through you.

6. Only use your cell phone to establish contact or for conversations lasting a few minutes, as the biological effects are directly related to the duration of exposure. For longer conversations, use a land line with a corded phone, not a cordless phone (which uses electromagnetic emitting technology similar to that of cell phones).

7. Switch sides regularly while communicating on your cell phone to spread out your exposure. Before putting your cell phone to the ear, wait until your correspondent has picked up. This limits the power of the electromagnetic field emitted near your ear and the duration of your exposure.

8. Avoid using your cell phone when the signal is weak or when moving at high speed, such as in a car or train, as this automatically increases power to a maximum as the phone repeatedly attempts to connect to a new relay antenna.

9. When possible, communicate via text messaging rather than making a call, limiting the duration of exposure and the proximity to the body.

10. Choose a device with the lowest SAR possible (SAR = Specific Absorption Rate, which is a measure of the strength of the magnetic field absorbed by the body). SAR ratings of contemporary phones by different manufacturers are available by searching for "sar ratings cell phones" on the internet.

Contact: upmc.com/Communications/MediaRelations

Publications

These resources are selected for their emphasis on natural approaches to issues of interest to our readers.

Anxiety and Obsessive Compulsive Disorder (OCD)

Anxious 9 to 5

Larina Kase; New Harbinger Publications 2006

A self-help book for adults offering cognitive-behavioral solutions for workplace anxiety—from doubting decisions to perfectionism, procrastination, public speaking anxiety, and fears of failure. Offers a strategy to beat anxiety and develop greater workplace confidence and success.

Freeing Your Child from Anxiety: Powerful, Practical Solutions to Overcome Your Child's Fears, Worries, and Phobias

Tamar E Chansky; Broadway Books/Random House 2004

A book for parents, therapists, and teachers which describes the basics of anxiety management and includes chapters on each anxiety disorder including separation anxiety, generalized anxiety, social anxiety, obsessive-compulsive disorder, panic disorder, and phobias. Also included are chapters on sleep issues, tics, habits, and hair-pulling.

Freeing Your Child from Obsessive-Compulsive Disorder: Powerful, Practical Strategies for Parents of Children and Adolescents

Tamar Chansky; Three Rivers Press 2001

Written for parents, therapists, and teachers, this book "cracks the code" of a confusing disorder and details the steps to take in tackling the four themes of OCD: contamination, checking/repeating/redoing, symmetry, and intrusive thoughts.

Attention Deficit Disorder/Hyperactivity (ADHD) and Behavior

ADD: The 20-Hour Solution

Mark Steinberg and Siegfried Othmer; Robert D. Reed Authors Choice Publishing 2004
The authors specialize in the use of EEG biofeedback techniques (also called neurofeedback) for the attention, behavior, mood, and learning problems of children and adults. Text provides a good framework for parents to understand the benefits of neurofeedback and how it works.

Biofeedback for the Brain: How Neurotherapy Effectively Treats Depression, ADHD, Autism, and More

Paul Swingle; Rutgers University Press 2008
Swingle's book has a focus on ADHD, employing a methodology he developed that is considered outside the traditional approach.

Crime Times

A free online newsletter on biological causes of behavioral and learning disorders, with research reviews of successful nutritional treatments. Published by the Wacker Foundation. crimetimes.org

Dr. Bob's Guide to Stop ADHD in 18 Days: Stop Medicating ADHD, ADD, OCD— Treat Hyperactivity Naturally!

Robert DeMaria; Drugless Healthcare Solutions, 2005
A quick-start guide to behavioral change. Diet is a main focus of the book with an emphasis on omega fatty acids. The role of parenting is highlighted.

No More ADHD: 10 Steps to Help Improve Your Child's Attention & Behavior without Drugs

Mary Ann Block; Block System 2001
A readable guide that covers the need for dietary change in ADHD, vitamin supplementation, the role of allergy and digestion in this disorder, and the value of osteopathic manipulation. Tips on searching for the cause of symptoms are included.

The ADD Answer: How to Help Your Child Now

Frank Lawlis; Penguin Group 2004
Dr. Frank Lawlis shows parents how to claim their role in healing their children with

step-by-step advice on dealing with the problems of ADD. His integrative approach explores the role of nutrition in treating the disorder, effects of counseling and goal setting, advances in the field of biofeedback, and environmental issues.

Why Can't My Child Behave?: Why Can't She Cope? Why Can't He Learn?

Jane Hersey; Pear Tree Press 1996

Hersey, director of the Feingold Association, prepared this guide to help parents understand and implement additive-free diets. While not a new offering, it contains time-tested approaches, and addresses common concerns and challenges for families seeking to improve behavior and health in their children through dietary change.

Autism

A Drug-Free Approach to Asperger Syndrome and Autism: Homeopathic Care for Exceptional Kids

Judyth Reichenberg-Ullman and Robert Ullman; Picnic Point Press 2005

The use of homeopathy is described by the authors, both leading naturopaths, as a treatment for children on the autism spectrum.

Autism: Effective Biomedical Treatments; Have We Done Everything We Can for this Child? 2007 Supplement

Jon Pangborn and Sidney Baker; Autism Research Institute 2007

This pamphlet-update is available from Autism Research International. It contains philosophical, scientific, and informational updates on the latest biomedical approaches to the diagnosis and treatment of autism, PDD, and related disorders. A "must have" companion text for the 2005 edition of *Autism: Effective Biomedical Treatments* also by Pangborn and Baker. The text is considered the manual for Defeat Autism Now! efforts.

Children with Starving Brains: A Medical Treatment Guide for Autism Spectrum Disorder 3rd edition

Jaquelyn McCandless; Bramble Books 2007

Dr. McCandless, active in the Defeat Autism Now! movement, was one of the first physicians to write a comprehensive and detailed guide on biomedical approaches to autism and related disorders. This latest edition includes cutting edge developments on numerous integrative approaches, including hyperbaric oxygen therapy.

Louder than Words: A Mother's Journey in Healing Autism

Jenny McCarthy; Plume; reprint edition 2008

Jenny McCarthy has gained national recognition for sharing her journey as she discovered an intense combination of behavioral therapy, diet, and supplements that became the key to saving her son from autism.

Recovering Autistic Children

Stephen Edelson and Bernard Rimland; Autism Research Institute 2006

This book is an extensively updated and enlarged revision of *Treating Autistic Children* (2003). It includes information from Autism Research Institute's Defeat Autism Now! project and new sections including clinical use of methyl-B$_{12}$, the specific carbohydrate diet, low-dose naltrexone, chelation, medical marijuana to control aggression, and more.

Depression

Dealing with Depression Naturally: Complementary and Alternative Therapies for Restoring Emotional Health

Syd Baumel; Keats Publishing 2000

A self-help guide, Baumel's well written text tells readers how to assess the pros and cons of natural therapies, from vitamins and dietary adjustments to visualization exercises and sleep therapy.

What Your Doctor May Not Tell You about Depression

Michael B Schachter with Deborah Mitchell; Wellness Central 2006

Dr. Schachter offers methods to treat depression naturally through rebalancing and repairing out-of-sync and inefficient neurotransmitters in the brain. Readers will learn how safe natural supplements and proper nutrition can directly affect brain chemistry, effectively controlling the amount of serotonin, dopamine, and glutamine in the brain without the use of drugs.

The Mood Cure: The 4-Step Program to Take Charge of Your Emotions—Today

Julia Ross; Penguin (Non-Classics) 2003

Ross provides a prescriptive plan designed to relieve a variety of ailments from seasonal disorders, stress, irritability, and depression through a change in diet and use of nutritional supplements. Readers are asked to first determine which of four "false moods" they suffer from: a dark cloud, blahs, stress, or too much sensitivity, through a survey in the book. Using survey scores, readers can then turn to the appropriate chapter to learn which diets and supplements could be most helpful.

Diet and Nutrition

Biochemical, Physiological & Molecular Aspects of Human Nutrition, 2nd Edition

Martha Stipanuk; Saunders 2006

A professional level textbook. This book presents advanced nutrition in a comprehensive, easy-to-understand format ideal for graduate students in nutritional programs, organic chemistry, physiology, biochemistry, and molecular biology. It focuses on the biology of human nutrition at the molecular, cellular, tissue, and whole-body levels. Includes student-friendly features such as chapter outlines, common abbreviations, critical thinking exercises, and detailed illustrations. Feature boxes spotlight key nutritional data, insights, and clinical correlations. Chapters are organized logically into seven units, reflecting the traditional nutrient class divisions.

Food Allergies and Food Intolerance: The Complete Guide to their Identification and Treatment

Jonathan Brostoff and Linda Gamlin; Healing Arts Press 2000

Brostoff, a researcher and international authority on food allergy, and Gamlin, a biochemist, clarify the difference between allergy and intolerance and identify common allergens and treatment options. A detailed elimination diet and reintroduction schedule is included.

Gluten-Free Quick & Easy: From Prep to Plate without the Fuss—200+ Recipes for People with Food Sensitivities

Carol Fenster; Avery 2007

The author reveals her time-saving tips and techniques to help cooks put homemade gluten-free meals on the table "in a flash." From entrees to desserts, this new book should help those trying to deal with cooking for special diets.

The Kid-Friendly ADHD & Autism Cookbook: The Ultimate Guide to the Gluten-Free, Casein-Free Diet

Pamela Compart and Dana Laake; Fair Winds Press 2006

Kid-friendly recipes and a guide to the gluten-free, milk-free diet. The book provides successful suggestions for feeding the picky eater. Specialty ingredients are explained and sources given, along with testimonials from parents and children.

Environmental Issues

Chemical-Free Kids: How to Safeguard Your Child's Diet and Environment

Allan Magaziner, Linda Bonvie, and Anthony Zolezzi; Twin Streams Books 2003

Learn how to phase out products that contain harmful additives and replace them with healthier ones without disrupting your lifestyle. Tips are given to protect your family, starting with pregnancy.

Growing Up Green: Baby and Child Care

Deirdre Imus; Simon & Schuster 2008

The second volume in the *New York Times* bestselling "Green This!" series, *Growing Up Green: Baby and Child Care* is a complete guide to raising healthy kids. Environmental activist and children's advocate Deirdre Imus addresses specific issues faced by children in every age group—from infants to adolescents and beyond. With a focus on preventing childhood illnesses, Imus concentrates on educating and empowering parents to recognize and avoid toxins that surround and endanger us all.

Healing the New Childhood Epidemics: Autism, ADHD, Asthma, and Allergies: The Ground-breaking Program for the 4-A Disorders

Kenneth Bock and Cameron Stauth; Ballantine Books 2008

Using the maxim: "genetics load the gun and environment pulls the trigger," the authors explain how heavy metals, exposure to viruses through vaccination, and poor nutrition create a harmful situation for children. Written as a guide for parents and professionals.

Is This Your Child?

Doris Rapp; Bantum Books 1997

A classic description of how environmental insults affect children, and how the negative impact on the immune system is often overlooked. See also Rapp's book: *Is This Your Child's World?*

Other

Alternative Therapies in Health and Medicine

Started in 1995, *Alternative Therapies in Health and Medicine* is a bi-monthly venue for sharing information on the use of alternative therapies in preventing and treating disease, healing illness, and promoting health. The magazine does not endorse any particular methodology, but promotes the evaluation and appropriate use of all effective approaches. The journal encourages the integration of alternative therapies with conventional medical practices. InnoVision Health Media, Inc.; alternative-therapies.com

Integrative Medicine: A Clinician's Journal

Launched as a peer-reviewed journal in 2002, articles provide practitioners with a practical and comprehensive approach to integrating alternative therapies with conventional medicine. The journal is published 6 times per year under the leadership of Joseph Pizzorno, ND, editor in chief, a co-founder and former president of Bastyr University; InnoVision Health Media, Inc.; imjournal.com

Natural Healing for Schizophrenia and Other Common Mental Disorders, Revised 3rd Edition

Eva Edelman; Borage Books 2001

Well researched and detailed, Edelman's excellent and ground-breaking text can be used as a treatment guide by professionals.

The Inflammation Cure

William Meggs with Carol Svec; McGraw Hill 2004

In clear, understandable language, the authors explain what causes inflammation, its relationship to disease in the body, and what steps readers can take to minimize their risk. Recommendations to reverse and avoid inflammation (which can affect the brain) are valuable.

Mothering: Natural Family Living

An established and reputable magazine sold online in digital format and in print version in stores and home delivery. From the kitchen to the environment, babies to parents, medical to social issues, an open-minded approach to new natural efforts is embraced. mothering.com

Natural Health Magazine

This magazine serves as a practical guide to good health. Each issue includes information on naturally-oriented food and nutrition, alternative health practices, exercise, and self-care. *Natural Health* focuses on the mind/body connection, illustrated exercise, preventative medicine, healthy cuisines, creating a healthy lifestyle in the home and office, and consumer guides to natural products. naturalhealthmag.com

The Out-of-Sync Child: Recognizing and Coping with Sensory Integration Dysfunction, *Revised Edition*

Carol Stock Kranowitz; Perigee Trade 2006

The Out-of-Sync Child broke new ground by identifying Sensory Processing Disorder, a common but frequently misdiagnosed problem in which the central nervous system misinterprets messages from the senses. This newly revised edition features additional information from recent research on vision and hearing deficits, motor skill problems, nutrition and picky eaters, ADHD, autism, and other related disorders.

PDR for Herbal Medicines, *4th Edition*

Joerg Gruenwald, Thomas Brendler, and Christof Jaenicke; Thomson Healthcare 2007

PDR has compiled a list of extensive explanations of more than 600 herbal medications available. Addressing the influx of natural supplements into mainstream supermarkets, PDR intends to educate consumers and assist them in choosing the best herbs to treat an ailment or simply to help maintain a healthy life. Each herbal entry contains pertinent information: description, physical properties, intended usage and expected effects, precautions and adverse reactions, recommended dosage, and references for additional reading. To assist in identifying these supplements, the editors have included color photos of many of these herbs as they exist naturally.

Townsend Letter: The Examiner of Alternative Medicine

Since 1983, *Townsend Letter* has been publishing a print alternative medicine magazine. Designed for the entire alternative medicine community, it presents scientific information (pro and con) on a wide variety of alternative medicine topics including EDTA chelation therapy; townsendletter.com

Tics and Tourette Syndrome (TS)

There Ain't No Can't: A Tribute to a Child's Struggle and Colossal Achievement

Jeffrey Feldstein; Avid Readers Publishing Group 2008

The author's son, Noah, was diagnosed with Tourette syndrome at an early age. With the help of an environmental physician, the family began specialized nutritional therapy with significant dietary changes to address food sensitivities. This effort, coupled with success strategies developed by Feldstein and detailed for the reader, resulted in excellent progress in symptom control.

Organizations

Acupuncture/Chinese Medicine

American Academy of Medical Acupuncture (AAMA)

The purpose of the AAMA is to promote the integration of traditional and modern forms of acupuncture with Western medical training in order to arrive at a more comprehensive approach to health care.

4929 Wilshire Boulevard, Suite 428

Los Angeles, CA 90010

323.937.5514

medicalacupuncture.org

American Association of Acupuncture and Oriental Medicine (AAAOM)

Provides information for practitioners of acupuncture and oriental medicine as well as students and patients. AAAOM seeks to integrate these disciplines into mainstream health care in the United States. It also aims to establish, maintain, and advance the profession as a distinct, primary care field of medicine.

PO Box 162340

Sacramento, CA 95816

916.443.4770; 866.455.7999

aaaomonline.org

Behavior and Cognitive Therapy

The Academy of Cognitive Therapy (ACT)

A non-profit mental health organization founded by experts in the field of cognitive therapy. Provides information as well as referrals for therapists in your area.

260 South Broad Street, 18th Floor

Philadelphia, PA 19102

610.664.1273

academyofct.org

Association for Behavioral and Cognitive Therapies (ABCT)

ABCT is an interdisciplinary organization committed to the advancement of human behavior through the investigation and application of behavioral, cognitive, and other evidence-based principles. Offers a practitioner referral list.

305 7th Avenue, 16th Floor
New York, NY 10001
212.647.1890
abct.org

Worry Wise Kids Website

The Children's Center for OCD and Anxiety, a behavioral treatment center under the direction of Tamar Chansky, PhD, sponsors the unique Worry Wise Kids website to help children cope with and overcome stress, worry, and anxieties in their life.

Children's Center for OCD and Anxiety
3138 Butler Pike
Plymouth Meeting, PA 19462
484.530.0778
worrywisekids.org

Biofeedback

Association for Applied Psychophysiology and Biofeedback (AAPB)

AAPB was founded 40 years ago as the Biofeedback Research Society. AAPB's mission is to advance the development, dissemination, and utilization of knowledge about applied psychophysiology and biofeedback to improve health and the quality of life through research, education, and practice. See Web site for publications, news, and a list of providers.

10200 W 44th Avenue, Suite 304
Wheat Ridge, CO 80033
303.422.8436; 800.477.8892
aapb.org

EEG Spectrum International, Inc.

EEG Spectrum International, Inc. is recognized within the neurofeedback community as being in the forefront of the field. It has more than 600 affiliates and associates worldwide and is assisting in research in the areas of autism, chemical sensitivity, and substance abuse, as well as optimal performance for nonclinical populations. Under the direction of Susan and Siegfried Othmer. it provides referrals, FAQs, and a wealth of information for the public and professionals.

21601 Vanowen Street, Suite 100

Canoga Park, CA 91303

818.789.3456

eegspectrum.com

Biomedical Approaches to Autism

Researchers, physicians, and families connected with autism spectrum disorders are making dramatic progress in developing biomedical approaches for these children that are reversing the symptoms. Many of the applications (such as preventive steps, dietary change, nutritional support, and detoxification) can be adapted for use with Tourette syndrome and related disorders. As such, readers are encouraged to stay abreast of developments in this field. The Autism Research Institute is highlighted below because, to a large degree, it is credited with the success of this movement. Several other important links that provide valuable information and/or services on biomedical treatments follow.

Autism Research Institute (ARI)

For more than 40 years, ARI, a non-profit organization, has devoted its work to disseminating the results of all related research, information on the triggers of autism, and on methods of diagnosing and treating autism. Through its Defeat Autism Now! program, ARI provides research-based information to parents, clinicians, and researchers worldwide.

4182 Adams Avenue

San Diego, CA 92116

866.366.3361

autism.com

Autism Society of America autism-society.org

Generation Rescue generationrescue.org

National Autism Association nationalautismassociation.org

Schafer Autism Report sarnet.org

AutismOne autismone.org

Medigenesis medigenesis.com

SafeMinds safeminds.org

Talk About Curing Autism talkaboutcuringautism.org

Unlocking Autism unlockingautism.org

Treating Autism treatingautism.org

Chiropractic medicine

American Chiropractic Association (ACA)

The American Chiropractic Association is the largest professional association in the world representing doctors of chiropractic. The ACA is involved with lobbying, public relations, professional and educational opportunities for doctors of chiropractic, research funding, and offers leadership for the advancement of the profession.
1701 Clarendon Blvd.
Arlington, VA 22209
703.276.8800
amerchiro.org

International Chiropractors Association (ICA)

Seeks to maintain and promote chiropractic's unique identity as a drugless and surgical-free health science, based on its fundamental principles and philosophy. It provides leadership in the establishment of chiropractic licensure regulation in every nation and promotes the quality and authenticity of chiropractic education. Provides international referrals.
1110 N Glebe Rd, Suite 650
Arlington, VA 22201
703.528.5000; 800.423.4690
chiropractic.org

Craniosacral Therapy

The Upledger Institute

The Upledger Institute, founded by John Upledger, DO, is a health resource center dedicated to the advancement of complementary and innovative techniques. It is recognized worldwide for its ground-breaking continuing education programs, clinical research, and therapeutic services. The institute offers hundreds of classes annually throughout North America, Central America, South America, Europe, India, Asia, the Middle East, New Zealand, and Australia. See the Web site for information on craniosacral therapy and related modalities, trainings, and practitioner referrals.

11211 Prosperity Farms Road, Suite D-325

Palm Beach Gardens, FL 33410

561.622.4334

upledger.com

Dental—holistic or biological

Holistic Dental Association (HDA)

Since 1978, HDA has been providing support and guidance to practitioners of holistic and alternative dentistry, as well as informing the public of the benefits of holistic dentistry for their health and well-being. Referrals provided.

PO Box 151444

San Diego, CA 92175

619.923.3120

holisticdental.org

International Academy of Oral Medicine & Toxicology (IAOMT)

The IAOMT is a network of dental, medical, and research professionals who seek to raise the standards of dental practice with information from the latest interdisciplinary research. In IAOMT sponsored conferences, lecturers are drawn from the field of medicine, physiology, toxicology, chemistry, biochemistry, risk and exposure assessment, materials science, immunology, microbiology, pharmacology, epidemiology, cardiology, neurology, nutrition, and other fields of science. Provides accreditation for practitioners and a referral service. A good source of information for families.

8297 ChampionsGate Blvd, #193

ChampionsGate, FL 33896

863.420.6373

iaomt.org

Diet Information

Center for Science in the Public Interest (CSPI)

Since 1971 CSPI has been a strong advocate for nutrition and health, food safety, alcohol policy, and sound science. Its award-winning newsletter, *Nutrition Action Healthletter,* with some 900,000 subscribers in the United States and Canada, is the largest-circulation health newsletter in North America.

1875 Connecticut Avenue NW, Suite 300

Washington, DC 20009

202.332.9110

Canada:

Suite 4550, CTTC Bldg.

1125 Colonel By Drive

Ottawa, Ontario K1S 5R1

613.244.7337

cspinet.org

Feingold Association of the United States (FAUS)

The Feingold Program (also known as the Feingold Diet) is a test to determine if certain foods or food additives are triggering particular symptoms. It is basically the way people used to eat before hyperactivity and ADHD became household words, and before asthma and chronic ear infections became common. The organization provides free information on the site and also has a paid membership and publication.

554 East Main Street, Suite 301

Riverhead, NY 11901

800.321.3287

feingold.org

Environmental & Green: Advocacy and Products

American Environmental Health Foundation

The American Environmental Health Foundation (AEHF) was founded in 1975 by William J Rea, MD of the Environmental Health Center: Dallas. An array of 1,500 environmentally friendly products and informative publications are available through the Web site. The products available on the AEHF Web site were designed to meet the needs of the chemically sensitive and environmentally aware individual.

8345 Walnut Hill Lane, Suite 225

Dallas, TX 75231

214.361.9515

aehf.com

Care2 Make a Difference

Care2 is a leading network of members with a focus on green living. Free environmental tips, networking, news, and products for purchase are available.

275 Shoreline Drive, Suite 300

Redwood City, CA 94065

650.622.0860

care2.com

Environmental Working Group (EWG)

EWG describes their staff as a team of scientists, engineers, policy experts, lawyers, and computer programmers that examines government data, legal documents, scientific studies, and EWG's laboratory tests to expose threats to health and the environment, and to find solutions. An exceptionally useful Web site.

1436 U Street NW, Suite 100

Washington, DC 20009

202.667.6982

ewg.org

Maine Organic Farmers and Gardeners Association (MOFGA)

MOFGA, formed in 1971, is the oldest and largest state organic organization in the country. Its goal is to help farmers and gardeners grow organic food, protect the environment, recycle natural resources, increase local food production, support rural communities, and educate consumers. Excellent Web site offers important information, publications, and resources.

PO Box 170

294 Crosby Brook Road

Unity, Maine 04988

207.568.4142

mofga.org

Microwave News

An online website with free news reports. For more than 25 years, *Microwave News* has been reporting on the potential health and environmental impacts of electromagnetic fields and radiation. The site is recognized as a fair and objective source of information. *Microwave News* is independent and is not aligned with any industry or government agency. The reports cover the nonionizing electromagnetic spectrum, with special emphasis on mobile phones and power lines, as well as radar and broadcast towers.

155 East 77th Street, Suite 3D
New York, NY 10075
212.517.2800
microwavenews.com

Nutritional Ecological Environmental Delivery System (NEEDS)

This international mail order resource specializes in providing products, information, and education in the areas of chemical sensitivity, environmental illness, fibromyalgia, celiac disease, and candida. Products include vitamins/supplements, environmental equipment (air and water purification, portable saunas, oral hygiene, seasonal affective disorder and electromagnetic field products), gluten-free foods, personal care items, domestic and pet care items, and a variety books.

6666 Manlius Center Road
East Syracuse, NY 13057
800.634.1380
needs.com

Organic Consumers Association (OCA)

OCA is an online and grassroots nonprofit organization campaigning for health, justice, and sustainability. The OCA deals with issues of food safety, industrial agriculture, genetic engineering, children's health, corporate accountability, Fair Trade, environmental sustainability and other topics. The OCA represents over 850,000 members, subscribers, and volunteers, including several thousand businesses.

6771 South Silver Hill Drive
Finland, MN 55603
218.226.4164
organicconsumers.org

Seventh Generation

A source of non-toxic household and personal care products that are readily available at natural food stores and many other outlets. Orders can also be placed online. Free newsletter.

60 Lake Street
Burlington, VT 05401
802.658.3773; 800.456.1191
seventhgeneration.com

Herbal Therapy

American Botanical Council (ABC)

ABC is directed by Mark Blumenthal, who also founded the organization. They are an independent, nonprofit research and education group dedicated to providing accurate and reliable information for consumers, healthcare practitioners, researchers, educators, industry, and the media on the responsible use of herbal medicine.

PO Box 144345
Austin, TX 78714-4345
512.926.4900
abc.herbalgram.org

Holistic and Related Medical Organizations

American Academy of Environmental Medicine (AAEM)

The specialty in medicine in which doctors assist patients in uncovering the cause and effect relationship between their environment and their ill-health, and help them learn to avoid those inciting factors, is called environmental medicine. AAEM was founded in 1965 and is an international association of physicians and other professionals interested in the clinical aspects of man and his environment. Practitioner referrals online.

6505 E. Central Avenue, #296
Wichita, KS 67206
316.684.5500
aaemonline.org

American Association of Integrative Medicine (AAIM)

Suggesting that "health is more than the absence of disease," AAIM encourages a multi-disciplinary approach to medicine. It is a gathering place for healers, educators, and researchers from all specialties to compare notes and combine forces, benefiting both the patient and the health care provider.

2750 East Sunshine
Springfield, MO 65804
417.881.9995
aaimedicine.com

American College for Advancement in Medicine (ACAM)

ACAM is a not-for-profit association dedicated to educating physicians and other health care professionals on the latest findings and emerging procedures in complementary, alternative, and integrative medicine. ACAM enables members of the public to connect with physicians who take an integrative approach to patient care and empowers people with information about integrative medicine treatment options. Referrals available.

24411 Ridge Route, Suite 115
Laguna Hills, CA 92653
949.309.3520
acam.org

British Holistic Medical Association

The BHMA is an open association of mainstream healthcare professionals, complementary and alternative practitioners, and members of the public who want to adopt a more holistic approach in their own life and work. They promote understanding of the science and application of the mind-body connection, and encourage integration of complementary and alternative medicine within the National Health Service in order to widen public and professional choice.

PO Box 371
Bridgwater
Somerset, TA6 9BG UK
+44(0)1278 722 000
bhma.org

HealthInsite

HealthInsite is an Australian Government initiative, funded by the Department of Health and Ageing. It aims to improve the health of Australians by providing easy access to quality information about human health. HealthInsite has a section that includes research on complementary and alternative therapies for mental health conditions. Go to the Web site below and search for "alternative therapies," then look for the areas you are interested in.

Department of Health and Ageing, MDP 2

GPO Box 9848

Canberra ACT 2601

02 6289 8488

healthinsite.gov.au

Health Research Institute & Pfeiffer Treatment Center

Pfeiffer Treatment Center (PTC) is a not-for-profit, medical outpatient facility specializing in the treatment of symptoms from biochemical imbalances. PTC's medical team treats children, teens, and adults with symptoms of behavioral and learning disorders, attention deficit disorders, autism spectrum disorders, depression, bipolar disorder, schizophrenia, anxiety, post traumatic stress syndrome, and Alzheimer's disease. PTC takes a unique, integrative approach to identify and treat the root metabolic causes of these symptoms with a multi-disciplinary clinical team involving physicians, nurses, dietitians, pharmacists, and other clinical specialists.

4575 Weaver Parkway

Warrenville, IL 60555-4039

630.505.0300; 866.504.6076

hriptc.org

Institute for Functional Medicine (IFM)

Functional medicine is patient-centered health care that addresses the unique interactions among genetic, environmental, and lifestyle factors influencing both health and complex, chronic disease. It includes the concept of biochemical individuality describes the importance of individual variations in metabolic function that derive from genetic and environmental differences among individuals. Check the Web site for upcoming conferences.

4411 Pt. Fosdick Drive NW, Suite 305

PO Box 1697
Gig Harbor, WA 98335
800.228.0622
functionalmedicine.org

International Society for Orthomolecular Medicine (ISOM)

Founded by Abram Hoffer, MD, ISOM educates health professionals and the public in the benefits and practice of orthomolecular (nutritional) medicine through publications, conferences, and seminars. Sign up online for free e-reports; subscription journal available.

16 Florence Avenue
Toronto, Ontario
Canada M2N 1E9
416.733.2117
orthomed.org

Safe Harbor

A large site on non-drug approaches for mental health with testimonials, over 100 articles, and a directory of alternative mental health practitioners. See the Web site for their bookstore, support groups, email lists, and free monthly newsletter.

787 W. Woodbury Rd. #2
Altadena, CA 91001
626.791.7868
alternativementalhealth.com

Homeopathy

American Institute of Homeopathy

An association of medical and osteopathic physicians, dentists, advanced practice nurses, and physician assistants dedicated to the practice, promotion, and improvement of homeopathic medicine.

801 N. Fairfax Street, Suite 306
Alexandria, VA 22314
888.445.9988
homeopathyusa.org

Massage

American Massage Therapy Association

Informative site with news, membership, massage schools, public information, and referrals.

500 Davis Street, Suite 900

Evanston, IL 60201-4695

847.864.0123; 877.905.2700

amtamassage.org

Naturopathic Therapy

American Association of Naturopathic Physicians (AANP)

The growing field of naturopathic medicine offers natural therapies as a vital part of health care systems. Memberships and referrals.

4435 Wisconsin Avenue, NW, Suite 403

Washington, DC 20016

202.237.8150; 866.538.2267

naturopathic.org

Osteopathy

The Cranial Academy (CA)

Cranial osteopathy is the study of anatomy and physiology of the cranium and its inter-relationship with the body as a whole. It may be applied for the prevention and treatment of disease and enhancement of health within the practice of the science of osteopathy. The mission of the international Cranial Academy, founded in 1947, is to teach, advocate, and advance osteopathy, including osteopathy in the cranial field.

8202 Clearvista Parkway #9-D

Indianapolis, IN 46256

317.594.0411

cranialacademy.org

Some of the authors and/or practitioners included in this book:

John Boyles, Jr, MD
Dayton Ear, Nose & Throat
Surgeons, Inc.
7076 Corporate Way
Centerville, OH 45459
937.434.0555

Dale Gieringer, PhD, Vice Ch
NORML and the NORML Fnd
1600 K Street, NW, Suite 501
Washington, DC 20006-2832
202.483.5500
norml.org

Helen Irlen, MA, LMFT, Director
Irlen Institute
5380 Village Road
Long Beach, CA 90808
562.496.2550
Irlen.com

Joseph Mercola, DO
Natural Health Center
3200 West Higgins Road
Hoffman Estates, IL 60169
847.252.4310
mercola.com

Siegfried Othmer, PhD, Chief Scientist
EEGinfo.com
22020 Clarendon Street, Suite 305
Woodland Hills, CA 91367
818.373.1334
eeginfo.com

Jon B Pangborn, PhD
Bionostics, Inc.,
42 W. 719 Bridle Court
St. Charles, IL 60175

Judith Reichenberg-Ullman
The Northwest Center for
Homeopathic Medicine
131 Third Avenue N
Edmonds, WA 98020
425.774.5599
drugfreeasperger.com

Albert F. Robbins, DO, MSPH
420 W. Hillsboro Blvd.
Deerfield Beach, FL 33441
954.421.1929
allergycenter.com

Sherry A. Rogers, MD
PO Box 2716
Syracuse, NY 13220
315.488.2856
prestigepublishing.com

Julia Ross, Director
Recovery Systems, Inc
147 Lomita Drive, Suite D
Mill Valley, CA 94941
415.383.3611
moodcure.com

Amy Rothenberg, ND
The New England School
of Homeopathy
356 Middle Street

Amherst, MA 01002
413.256.5949
nesh.com

William Shaw, PhD
The Great Plains Laboratory, Inc.
11813 West 77th Street
Lenexa, KS 66214
913.341.8949
greatplainslaboratory.com

Vijendra K Singh, PhD
Department of Biology &
Biotechnology Center
Utah State University
5305 Old Main Hill
Logan, UT 84322

Tipu Sultan, MD
Environmental Health and
Allergy Center
11585 W Florissant Avenue
Florissant, MO 63033
314.921.5600
ehacstl.com

James W. Willoughby II, DO
24 S Main St.
Liberty, MO 64068
816.781.0902

Joseph S Wojcik, MD
525 Bronxville Road, Suite 1-G
Bronxville, NY 10708-1136
914.793.6161

SELECTED REFERENCES

Introduction and Chapter 1

1) Ananth J, Burgoyne KS, Niz D, Smith M: J Tardive dyskinesia in 2 patients treated with ziprasidone. *Psychiatry Neurosci* 2004;29:467-9.

2) Andrews N, Miller E, Grant A et al: Thimerosal exposure in infants and developmental disorders: a retrospective cohort study in the United Kingdom does not support a causal association. *Pediatrics* 2004;114:584-91.

3) Awaad Y: Tics in Tourette syndrome: new treatment options. *J Child Neurol* 1999;14:316-9.

4) Banaschewski T, Woerner W, Rothenberger A: Premonitory sensory phenomena and suppressibility of tics in Tourette syndrome: developmental aspects in children and adolescents. *Dev Med Child Neurol* 2003;45:700-3.

5) Bharucha KJ, Sethi KD: Tardive tourettism after exposure to neuroleptic therapy. *Mov Disord* 1995;10:791-3.

6) Comings DE: Clinical and molecular genetics of ADHD and Tourette syndrome. Two related polygenic disorders. *Ann N Y Acad Sci* 2001;931:50-83.

7) Eapen V, Robertson MM, Zeitlin H, Kurlan R: Gilles de la Tourette's syndrome in special education schools: a United Kingdom study. *J Neurol* 1997;244:378-82.

8) Frank MS, Sieg KG, Gaffney GR: Somatic complaints in childhood tic disorders. *Psychosomatics* 1991; 32:396-9.

9) Golden GS: The relationship between stimulant medication and tics. *Pediatr Ann* 1988;17:405-8.

10) Hershey T, Black KJ, Hartlein JM et al: Cognitive-pharmacologic functional magnetic resonance imaging in tourette syndrome: a pilot study. *Biol Psychiatry* 2004;55:916-25.

11) Ho CS, Shen EY, Shyur SD, Chiu NC: Association of allergy with Tourette's syndrome. *J Formos Med Assoc* 1999;98:492-5.

12) Howson AL, Batth S, Ilivitsky V et al: Clinical and attentional effects of acute nicotine treatment in Tourette's syndrome. *Eur Psychiatry* 2004;9:102-12.

13) Hyde TM, Emsellem HA, Randolph C, Rickler KC, Weinberger DR: Electroencephalographic abnormalities in monozygotic twins with Tourette's syndrome. *Br J Psychiatry* 1994;164:811-7.

14) Hyde TM, Weinberger DR: Tourette's syndrome. A model neuropsychiatric disorder. *JAMA* 1995;273:498-501.

15) Jankovic J: Medical Progress: Tourette's Syndrome. *N Engl J Med* 2001;345(16):1184-1192.

16) Kessler AR: Tourette syndrome associated with body temperature dysregulation: possible involvement of an idiopathic hypothalamic disorder. *J Child Neurol* 2002;17:738-44.

17) Khalifa N, von Knorring AL: Prevalence of tic disorders and Tourette syndrome in a Swedish school population. *Dev Med Child Neurol* 2003;45:315-9.

18) Kurlan R: Tourette's syndrome: are stimulants safe? *Curr Neurol Neurosci Rep* 2003;3:285-8.

19) Kurlan R, McDermott MP, Deeley C et al: Prevalence of tics in schoolchildren and association with place-

ment in special education. *Neurology* 2001;57:1383-88.

20) Kwak C, Vuong KD, Jankovic J: Migraine headache in patients with Tourette syndrome. *Arch Neurol* 2003;60:1595-8.

21) Leckman JF: Tourette's syndrome. *Lancet* 2002;360:1577-86.

22) Leckman JF, Zhang H, Vitale A et al: Course of tic severity in Tourette syndrome: the first two decades. *Pediatrics* 1998;102:14-19.

23) Lombroso PJ, Mack G, Scahill L, King RA, Leckman JF: Exacerbation of Gilles de la Tourette's syndrome associated with thermal stress: a family study. *Neurology* 1991;41:1984-7.

24) Mantel BJ, Meyers A, Tran QY, Rogers S, Jacobson JS: Nutritional supplements and complementary/alternative medicine in Tourette syndrome. *J Child Adolesc Psychopharmacol* 2004;14:582-9.

25) Marras C, Andrews D, Sime E, Lang AE: Botulinum toxin for simple motor tics: a randomized, double-blind, controlled clinical trial. *Neurology* 2001;56:605-10.

26) Mejia NI, Jankovic J: Secondary tics and tourettism. *Rev Bras Psiquiatr* 2005;27:11-7. E-pub.

27) Morshed SA, Parveen S, Leckman, JF et al: Antibodies against neural, nuclear, cytoskeletal, and streptococcal epitopes in children and adults with Tourette's syndrome, Ssenham's chorea, and autoimmune disorders. *Biological Psychiatry* 2001;50:566-77.

28) Muller-Vahl KR: Cannabinoids reduce symptoms of Tourette's syndrome. *Expert Opin Pharmacother* 2003; 4:1717-25.

29) Muller-Vahl KR, Schneider U, Koblenz A et al: Treatment of Tourette's syndrome with Delta 9-tetrahydrocannabinol (THC): a randomized crossover trial. *Pharmacopsychiatry* 2002;35:57-61.

30) Palumbo D, Spencer T, Lynch J, Co-Chien H, Faraone SV: Emergence of tics in children with ADHD: impact of once-daily OROS methylphenidate therapy *J Child Adolesc Psychopharmacol* 2004;14:185-94.

31) Peterson BS, Thomas P, Kane MJ et al: Basal Ganglia volumes in patients with Gilles de la Tourette syndrome. *Arch Gen Psychiatry* 2003;60:415-24.

32) Porta M, Maggioni G, Ottaviani F, Schindler A: Treatment of phonic tics in patients with Tourette's syndrome using botulinum toxin type A. *Neurol Sci* 2004;24:420-3.

33) Pringsheim T, Davenport WJ, Lang A: Tics. *Curr Opin Neurol* 2003;16: 523-7.

34) Randolph C, Hyde TM, Gold JM, Goldberg TE, Weinberger DR: Tourette's syndrome in monozygotic twins. Relationship of tic severity to neuropsychological function. *Arch Neurol* 1993;50:725-8.

35) Scahill L, Lombroso PJ, Mack G et al: Thermal sensitivity in Tourette syndrome: preliminary report. *Percept Mot Skills* 2001;92:419-32.

36) Singer HS: The treatment of tics. *Curr Neurol Neurosci Rep* 2001;1:195-202.

37) Snider LA, Seligman LD, Ketchen BR: Tics and problem behaviors in schoolchildren: prevalence, characterization, and associations. *Pediatrics* 2002;110:331-6.

38) Silva RR, Munoz DM, Barickman J, Friedhoff AJ: Environmental factors and related fluctuation of symptoms in children and adolescents with Tourette's disorder. *J Child Psychol Psychiatry* 1995;36:305-12.

39) Silver AA, Shytle RD, Philipp MK et al: Transdermal nicotine and haloperidol in Tourette's disorder: a double-blind placebo-controlled study. *J Clin Psychiatry* 2001;62:707-14.

40) Snider LA, Lougee L, Slattery M, Grant P, Swedo SE: Antibiotic prophylaxis with azithromycin or penicillin for childhood-onset neuropsychiatric disorders. *Biol Psychiatry* 2005;57:788-92.

41) Snider LA, Swedo SE. PANDAS: current status and directions for research. *Mol Psychiatry* 2004;9:900-7.

42) Straus SM, Bleumink GS, Dieleman JP et al: Antipsychotics and the risk of sudden cardiac death. *Arch Intern Med* 2004;164:1293-7.

43) Swedo SE: Pediatric autoimmune neuropsychiatric disorders associated with streptococcal infections (PANDAS). *Mol Psychiatry* 2002;7(suppl 2):S24-25.

44) Swedo SE, Grant PJ: Annotation: PANDAS: a model for human autoimmune disease. J *Child Psychol Psychiatry* 2005;46:227-34.

45) Swedo S, Leonard HL, Garvey M et al: Pediatric autoimmune neuropsychiatric disorders associated with streptococcal infection: clinical descriptions of the first 50 cases. *Am J Psychiatry*. 1998;155:264-271.

46) Tourette's Syndrome Study Group: Treatment of ADHD in children with tics: A randomized controlled trial. *Neurology* 2002;58:527-36.

47) Tourette Syndrome Assocation International Consortium for Genetics: *Am J Med Genet B Neuropsychiatr Genet* 2003;116(1):60-8.

48) Varley CK, Vincent J, Varley P, Calderon R: Emergence of tics in children with attention deficit hyperactivity disorder treated with stimulant medications. *Compr Psychiatry* 2001;42:228-33.

Chapter 3

1) Agency for Toxic Substances and Disease Registry. Toxicological profile for mercury. Atlanta, GA: US Department of Health and Human Services, March 1999.

2) Baldo JV, Ahmad L, Ruff R: Neuropsychological performance of patients following mold exposure. *Appl Neuropsychol* 2002;9:193-202.

3) Coffey BJ, Biederman J, Smoller JW et al: Anxiety disorders and tic severity in juveniles with Tourette's disorder. *J Am Acad Child Adolesc Psychiatry* 2000;39(5):562-8.

4) Cohrs S, Rasch T, Altmeyer S et al: Decreased sleep quality and increased sleep related movements in patients with Tourette's syndrome. *J Neurol Neurosurg Psychiatry* 2001;70(2):192-7.

5) Comings DE, Comings BG: A controlled study of Tourette syndrome. VI. Early development, sleep problems, allergies, and handedness. *Am J Hum Genet* 1987;41:822-38.

6) Feldman RG, Chirico-Post J, Proctor SP. Blink reflex latency after exposure to trichloroethylene in well water. *Arch Environ Health* 1988;43:143-8.

7) Gerr F, Letz R, Ryan PB, Green RC: Neurological effects of environmental exposure to arsenic in dust and soil among humans. *Neurotoxicology* 2000;21:475-87.

8) Gerrard JW, Richardson JS, Donat J: Neuropharmacological evaluation of movement disorders that are adverse reactions to specific foods. *Int. Journal of Neuroscience* 1994;76:61-9.

9) Hyde TM, Emsellem HA, Randolph C et al: Electroencephalographic abnormalities in monozygotic twins with Tourette's syndrome *Br J Psychiatry* 1994;164:811-7.

10) Frank MS, Sieg KG, Gaffney GR: Somatic complaints in childhood tic disorders. *Psychosomatics* 1991;32:396-9.

11) Finegold I: Allergy and Tourette's syndrome. A*nn Allergy* 1985;55:119-21.

12) Ho CS, Shen EY, Shyur SD, Chiu NC: Association of allergy with Tourette's syndrome. *J Formos Med Assoc* 1999;98:492-5.

13) Howson AL, Batth S, Ilivitsky V et al: Clinical and attentional effects of acute nicotine treatment in Tourette's syndrome. *Eur Psychiatry* 2004;9:102-12.

14) Kim H, Moote W, Mazza J: Tourette's syndrome in patients referred for allergy evaluation. *Ann Allergy Asthma Immunol* 1997;79:347-9.

15) Palumbo D, Spencer T, Lynch J, Co-Chien H, Faraone SV: Emergence of tics in children with ADHD: impact of once-daily OROS methylphenidate therapy. *J Child Adolesc Psychopharmacol* 2004;14:185-94.

16) Schober S, Sinks T, Jones R et al: Blood mercury levels in US children and women of childbearing age, 1999-2000. *JAMA* 2003;289:1667-74.

17) Silva RR, Munoz DM, Barickman J, Friedhoff AJ: Environmental factors and related fluctuation of symptoms in children and adolescents with Tourette's disorder. *J Child Psychol Psychiatry*. 1995;36:305-12.

18) Speer, Frederic, *Handbook of Clinical Allergy,* John Wright, Boston, London 1982.

19) Stern A, Smith A: An assessment of the cord blood:maternal blood methylmercury ratio: implications for risk assessment. *Environ Health Perspect* 2003;111:1465-70.

20) Tourette Syndrome Assocation International Consortium for Genetics: *Am J Med Genet B Neuropsychiatr Genet* 2003;116(1):60-8.

Chapter 9

1) Attias J, Sapir S, Bresloff I, Reshef-Haran I, Ising H: Reduction in noise-induced temporary threshold shift in humans following oral magnesium intake. *Clin Otolaryngol Allied Sci* 2004;29:635-41.
2) Ayres, A J: *Sensory Integration and the Child* 1979; Los Angeles: Western Psych. Services.
3) Barabas G, Matthews WS: Homogeneous clinical subgroups in children with Tourette syndrome. *Pediatrics* 1985;75:73-5.
4) Case-Smith J, Bryan T: The effects of occupational therapy with sensory integration emphasis on pre-school-age children with autism. *Am J Occup Ther* 1999.
5) Cevette MJ, Vormann J, Franz K: Magnesium and hearing. *J Am Acad Audiol* 2003;14:202-12.
6) Duggal HS, Nizamie SH: Bereitschaftspotential in tic disorders: a preliminary observation. *Neurol India* 2002;50:487-9.
7) Galland L: Magnesium, stress and neuropsychiatric disorders. *Magnes Trace Elem* 1991-92;10:287-301.
8) Hoehn, TP, Baumeister AA: A critique of the application of sensory integration therapy to children with learning disabilities. *Journal of Learning Disabilities* 1994, 27, 338-50.
9) Kranowitz CS, Silver LB: *The Out-of-Sync Child* 1998; New York: Peregree.
10) Leckman JF, Walker DE, Goodman WK, Pauls DL, Cohen DJ: "Just right" perceptions associated with compulsive behavior in Tourette's syndrome. *Am J Psychiatry* 1994;151:675-80.
11) Lombroso PJ, Mack G, Scahill L, King RA, Leckman JF: Exacerbation of Gilles de la Tourette's syndrome associated with thermal stress: a family study. *Neurology* 1991;41:1984-7.
12) Miguel EC, do Rosario-Campos MC, Prado HS et al: Sensory phenomena in obsessive-compulsive disorder and Tourette's disorder. *J Clin Psychiatry* 2000;61:150-6.
13) Rimland B, Edelson SM: Auditory Integration Training: Sound sensitivity in autism, Berard vs Tomatis approach. Autism Research Institute 2004; *www.autism.com/ari.*
14) Sachdev PS, Chee KY, Aniss AM: The audiogenic startle reflex in Tourette's syndrome. *Biol Psychiatry* 1997;41:796-803.
15) Sammeth CA, Preves DA, Brandy WT: Hyperacusis: case studies and evaluation of electronic loudness suppression devices as a treatment approach. *Scand Audiol* 2000;29:28-36.
16) Scahill L, Lombroso PJ, Mack G et al: Thermal sensitivity in Tourette syndrome: preliminary report. *Percept Mot Skills* 2001;92:419-32.
17) Schaaf RC, Miller LJ: Occupational therapy using a sensory integrative approach for children with developmental disabilities. *Ment Retard Dev Disabil Res Rev* 2005;11:143-8.
18) Shaw SR: A school psychologist investigates sensory integration therapies: promise, possibility, and the art of placebo; *NASP Communiqué* October 2002.
19) Sinha Y, Silove N, Wheeler D, Williams K: Auditory integration training and other sound therapies for autism spectrum disorders. *Cochrane Database Syst Rev* 2004;CD003681.

Chapter 10

1) Christakis DA, Zimmerman FJ, DiGiuseppe DL, McCarty CA: Early television exposure and subsequent attentional problems in children. *Pediatrics* 2004;113:708-13.
2) Dursun SM, Burke JG, Reveley MA: Antisaccade eye movement abnormalities in Tourette syndrome: evidence for cortico-striatal network dysfunction? *J Psychopharmacol* 2000;14:37-9.
3) Enoch JM, Itzhaki A, Lakshminarayanan V, Comerford JP et al: Visual field defects detected in patients

with Gilles de la Tourette syndrome: preliminary report. *Int Ophthalmol* 1989;13:331-44.

4) Enoch JM, Lakshminarayanan V, Itzhaki A et al: Anomalous kinetic visual fields found in family members of patients with a confirmed diagnosis of Gilles de la Tourette syndrome. *Optom Vis Sci* 1991;68:807-12.

5) Evans BJ, Busby A, Jeanes R, Wilkins AJ: Optometric correlates of Meares-Irlen syndrome: a matched group study. *Ophthalmic Physiol Opt* 1995;15:481-7.

6) Gobba F: Color vision: a sensitive indicator of exposure to neurotoxins. *Neurotoxicology* 2000;21:857-62.

7) Gobba F, Cavalleri A: Color vision impairment in workers exposed to neurotoxic chemicals. *Neurotoxicology* 2003;24:693-702.

8) Good PA, Taylor RH, Mortimer MJ: The use of tinted glasses in childhood migraine. *Headache* 1991;31:533-6.

9) Iregren A, Andersson M, Nylen P: Color vision and occupational chemical exposures: I. An overview of tests and effects. *Neurotoxicology* 2002;23:719-33.

10) Irlen, Helen: *Reading by the colors.* New York 1991; Avery.

11) Jeanes R, Busby A, Martin J, Lewis E et al: Prolonged use of coloured overlays for classroom reading. *Br J Psychol* 1997;88:531-48.

12) Lightstone A, Lightstone T, Wilkins A: Both coloured overlays and coloured lenses can improve reading fluency, but their optimal chromaticities differ. *Ophthalmic Physiol Opt* 1999;19:279-85.

13) Lombroso PJ, Mack G, Scahill L, King RA, Leckman JF: Exacerbation of Gilles de la Tourette's syndrome associated with thermal stress: a family study. *Neurology* 1991;41:1984-7.

14) Melun JP, Morin LM, Muise JG, DesRosiers M: Color vision deficiencies in Gilles de la Tourette syndrome. *J Neurol Sci* 2001;186:107-10.

15) Rea WJ, Didriksen N, Simon TR: Effects of toxic exposure to molds and mycotoxins in building-related illnesses. *Arch Environ Health* 2003;58:399-405.

16) Rice DC, Gilbert SG: Early chronic low-level methylmercury poisoning in monkeys impairs spatial vision. *Science* 1982;216:759-61.

17) Scahill L, Lombroso PJ, Mack G: Thermal sensitivity in Tourette syndrome: preliminary report. *Percept Mot Skills* 2001;92:419-32.

18) Solan HA, Ficarra A, Brannan JR, Rucker F: Eye movement efficiency in normal and reading disabled elementary school children: effects of varying luminance and wavelength. *J Am Optom Assoc* 1998;69:455-64.

19) Tatlipinar S, Iener EC, Ilhan B, Semerci B: Ophthalmic manifestations of Gilles de la Tourette syndrome. Eur J Ophthalmol 2001;11:223-6.

20) Urban P, Gobba F, Nerudova J et al: Color discrimination impairment in workers exposed to mercury vapor. *Neurotoxicology* 2003;24(4-5):711-6.

21) Utgard NA: Pineal melatonin in Tourette syndrome—can coloured light help? *Tidsskr Nor Laegeforen*;113:2420-1.

22) Whiting P, Robinson GL, Parrot CF: Irlen coloured filters for reading: A six year follow up. *Australian Journal of Remedial Education* 1994;26,13-19.

23) Wilkins AJ, Baker A, Amin D, Smith S et al: Treatment of photosensitive epilepsy using coloured glasses. *Seizure* 1999;8:444-9.

24) Zinner, Samuel H: Tourette syndrome—much more than tics. *Contemporary Pediatrics* 2004,Vol.21,No.8.

Chapter 11

1) Balikci K, Cem Ozcan I, Turgut-Balik D, Balik HH: A survey study on some neurological symptoms and sensations experienced by long term users of mobile phones. *Pathol Biol* 2005;53:30-4.

2) Barteri M, Pala A, Rotella S: Structural and kinetic effects of mobile phone microwaves on acetylcholinesterase activity. *Biophys Chem* 2005;113:245-53.

3) Bortkiewicz A, Zmyslony M, Szyjkowska A, Gadzicka E: Subjective symptoms reported by people living in

the vicinity of cellular phone base stations: review. *Med Pr* 2004;55:345-51.

4) Fejes I, Za Vaczki Z, Szollosi J et al: Is there a relationship between cell phone use and semen quality? *Arch Androl* 2005;51:385-93.

5) Firstenberg, A: Electromagnetic Fields (EMF) Killing Fields. *The Ecologist* 2004;vol 34:5.

6) Kavet R, Zaffanella LE: Contact voltage measured in residences: implications to the association between magnetic fields and childhood leukemia. *Bioelectromagnetics* 2002;23:464-74.

7) Kundi M, Mild K, Hardell L, Mattsson MO: Mobile telephones and cancer—a review of epidemiological evidence. *J Toxicol Environ Health B Crit Rev* 2004;7:351-84.

8) Scassellati-Sforzolini G, Moretti M, Villarini M et al: Evaluation of genotoxic and/or co-genotoxic effects in cells exposed in vitro to extremely-low frequency electromagnetic fields *Ann Ig* 2004;16:321-40.

Chapter 12

1) Andrews N, Miller E, Grant A et al: Thimerosal exposure in infants and developmental disorders: a retrospective cohort study in the United kingdom does not support a causal association. *Pediatrics* 2004;114:584-91.

2) Anthony H, Birtwistle S, Eaton K, Maberly J: *Environmental Medicine in Clinical Practice*, Southampton, 1997 BSAENM Publications.

3) Campbell AW, Thrasher JD, Madison RA et al: Neural autoantibodies and neurophysiologic abnormalities in patients exposed to molds in water-damaged buildings. *Arch Environ Health* 2003;58:464-74.

4) Cinca I, Dumitrescu I, Onaca P, Serbanescu A, Nestorescu B: Accidental ethylmercury poisoning with nervous system, skeletal muscle, and myocardium injury. *J Neurol Neurosurg Psychiatry* 1980;43:143-9.

5) Geier D, Geier MR: Neurodevelopmental disorders following thimerosal-containing childhood immunizations: a follow-up analysis. *Int J Toxicol* 2004;23:369-76.

6) Holmes AS, Blaxill MF, Haley BE: Reduced levels of mercury in first baby haircuts of autistic children. *Int J Toxic* 2003;22:277-85.

7) Horvath K, Papadimitriou J, Rabsztyn A, Drachenberg C, Tildon JT: Gastrointestinal abnormalities in children with autistic disorder. *J Ped* 1999;135:559-63.

8) Hyde TM, Emsellem HA, Randolph C, Rickler KC, Weinberger DR: Electroencephalographic abnormalities in monozygotic twins with Tourette's syndrome. *Br J Psychiatry.* 1994;164:811-7.

9) Hyde TM, Weinberger DR. Tourette's syndrome: A model neuropsychiatric disorder. *JAMA* 1995;273:498-501.

10) Kirby, David: *Evidence of Harm Mercury in Vaccines and the Autism Epidemic: A Medical Controversy.* New York, 2005, St Martin's Press.

11) Magaziner A, Bonvie L, Zolezzi A: *Chemical-Free Kids, How to Safeguard Your Child's Diet and Environment.* New York, 2003, Twin Streams, Kensington Publishing Corp.

12) Randolph C, Hyde TM, Gold JM, Goldberg TE, Weinberger DR: Tourette's syndrome in monozygotic twins. Relationship of tic severity to neuropsychological function. *Arch Neurol* 1993;50:725-8.

13) Rapp, Doris J: *Is This Your Child? Discovering and Treating Unrecognized Allergies in Children and Adults.* New York, 1991, William Morrow and Company.

14) Rapp, Doris J: *Our Toxic World, A Wake-Up Call.* Buffalo, 2005, Environmental Medical Research Foundation.

15) Rapp, Doris J: *Is This Your Child's World? How You Can Fix the Schools and Homes That Are Making Your Children Sick.* Bantam Books, 1996.

16) Rea WJ, Didriksen N, Simon TR: Effects of toxic exposure to molds and mycotoxins in building-related illnesses. *Arch Environ Health* 2003;58:399-405.

17) Silva RR, Munoz DM, Barickman J, Friedhoff AJ: Environmental factors and related fluctuation of symptoms in children and adolescents with Tourette's disorder. *J Child Psychol Psychiatry* 1995;36:305-12.

18) Snider LA, Seligman LD, Ketchen BR et al: Tics and problem behaviors in schoolchildren: prevalence, characterization, and associations. *Pediatrics* 2002;110:331-6.

19) Uchida T, Naito S, Kato H et al: Thimerosal induces toxic reaction in non-sensitized animals. *Int Arch Allergy Immunol* 1994;104:296-301.

20) Verstraeten T, Davis RL, DeStefano F et al: Vaccine Safety Datalink Team. Safety of thimerosal-containing vaccines: a two-phased study of computerized health maintenance organization databases. *Pediatrics* 2003;112:1039-48.

21) Wakefield AJ, Anthony A, Murch SH, Thomson M, Montgomery SM, Davis S et al: Enterocolitis in children with developmental disorders. A*m J Gastroenterol* 2000;95:2285-95.

22) Wigle, DT: *Child Health and the Environment,* New York, 2003, Oxford University Press.

Chapter 14

1) Ashford N, Miller C: *Chemical Exposures, Low Levels and High Stakes*, Second Edition, New York, 1998, Van Nostrand Reinhold.

2) Brennan, James C: *Basics of Food Allergy*, Second Edition, Springfield, Illinois 1984, Charles Thomas Publisher.

3) Brostoff, Jonathan: *Food Allergy and Intolerance,* London, 1987, Bailliere Tindall.

4) Comings, David E: *Search for the Tourette Syndrome and Human Behavior Genes*, Durarte, California, 1996, Hope Press.

5) Gerrard JW, Richardson JS, Donat J: Neuropharmacological evaluation of movement disorders that are adverse reactions to specific foods. *Int Journal of Neuroscience* 1994;76:61-9.

6) Ho CS, Shen EY, Shyur SD, Chiu NC: Association of allergy with Tourette's syndrome. *J Formos Med Assoc* 1999;98:492-5.

7) Hyde TM, Weinberger DR: Tourette's syndrome: A model neuropsychiatric disorder. *JAMA* 1995;273:498-501.

8) Introduction to Indoor Air Quality, A Reference Manual, July 1997, EPA #400/3-91/003.

9) King H: *Otolaryngic Allergy*, New York 1981, Symposia Specialists, Inc.

10) Kronse H: *Otolaryngic Allergy and Immunology*, Philadelphia, 1989, WB Saundrees Co.

11) Miller JB: *Relief at Last, Neutralization for Food Allergy and other Illnesses*, Springfield, Illinois, 1987, Charles Thomas Publisher.

12) Rea W: *Chemical Sensitivity,* Vols 1 through 4, 1995, Boca Raton, Florida, CRC Press.

13) Robbins AF: Chemically Induced Illness, pts 1 and 2. *Osteopathic Medical News,* September and October 1989.

14) Rom WN: *Environmental and Occupational Medicine,* Third Edition, Philadelphia 1998, Lippincott-Raven.

15) Speer F: *Handbook of Clinical Allergy*, Boston, London 1982, John Wright.

16) Tarcher A: *Principals and Practice of Environmental Medicine*, New York and London, 1992, Plenum Medical Book Co.

Chapter 15

1) Singh VK: Immunotherapy for brain diseases and mental illnesses. *Prog Drug Res* 1997;48:129-146.

2) Singh VK: Neuroautoimmunity: Pathogenic implications for Alzheimer's disease. *Gerontology* 1997;43:79-94.

3) Singh VK: Neuro-immunopathogenesis in autism. *New Frontier of Biology* (edited by Berczi I, Gorczynski RM), The Netherlands, 2001;443-454. Elsevier Science BV, Inc.

4) Singh VK, Rivas WH: Prevalence of serum antibodies to caudate nucleus in autistic children. *Neurosci Lett* 2004;355:53-56.

5) Trifiletti RR, Bandele AN: Serum antibodies to specific brain proteins in children with tics, Tourette's syndrome, or obsessive-compulsive disorder. *Ann Neurol* 2000;48:511-512.

6) Leckman JF , Katsovich L, Kawikova I et al: Increased serum levels of interleukin-12 and tumor necrosis factor-alpha in Tourette's syndrome. *Biol Psychiatry* 2005;57:667-673.

7) Singh, VK: Cytokine Regulation in autism. *Cytokines and Mental Health* (edited by Ziad Kronfol), pp 369-83, 2003, Boston, Kluwer Academic Publishers.

8) Singh, VK, Lin SX, Newell E, Nelson C: Abnormal measles virus serology and CNS autoimmunity in children with autism. *J Biomed Sci* 2002;461:359-64.

9) Singh, VK, Jensen, R: Elevated levels of measles antibodies in children with autism. *Pediatr Neurol* 2003;28:292-4.

10) Singh, VK, Rivas WH: Detection of antinuclear and antilaminin antibodies in autistic children who received thimerosal-containing vaccines. *J Biomed Sci* 2004;11:607-10.

11) Singh VK, Singh EA, Warren RP: Hyperserotoninemia and serotonin receptor antibodies in children with autism but not mental retardation. *Biol Psychiatry* 1997;41:753-5.

12) Hanna GL, Singh VK, Curtis GC et al: Serotonin receptor antibodies in early-onset obsessive-compulsive disorder. Proceedings of the 43rd Annual Meeting of the American Academy of Child and Adolescent Psychiatry 1996; Philadelphia, Pennsylvania; October 10-15.

13) Perlmutter SJ, Leitman SF, Garvey MA: Therapeutic plasma exchange and intravenous immunoglobulin for obsessive-compulsive disorder and tic disorders in children. *Lancet* 1999;354:1153-8.

14) Singh VK: Rehabilitation of autism with immune modulation therapy. *Journal of Special Education and Rehabilitation* 2004;3-4:161-78.

Chapter 16

1) Alberti A, Pirrone P, Elia M et al: Sulphation deficit in "low-functioning" autistic children: a pilot study. *Biological Psychiatry* 1999;46:420-4.

2) Aydogan B, Kiroglu M, Altintas D et al: The role of food allergy in otitis media with effusion. *Otolaryngol Head Neck Surg* 2004;130:747-50.

3) Bateman BJ, Warner JO, Hutchinson E et al: The effects of a double blind, placebo controlled, artificial food colourings and benzoate preservative challenge on hyperactivity in a general population sample of preschool children. *Archives of Disease in Childhood* 2004;89:506-11.

4) Baylock RL: *Excitotoxins, the Taste that Kills*, Santa Fe, 1997, Health Press.

5) Bell W, Clapp R, Davis D et al: Carcinogenicity of saccharin in laboratory animals and humans: letter to Dr. Harry Conacher of Health Canada. *Int J Occup Environ Health* 2002;8:387-93.

6) Briffa J: Aspartame and its effects on health: independently funded studies have found potential for adverse effects. *BMJ* 2005;330:309-10.

7) Butchko HH, Stargel WW, Comer CP et al: Aspartame: review of safety. *Regul Toxicol Pharmacol* 2002;35:S1-93.

8) Camfield PR, Camfield CS, Dooley JM et al: Aspartame exacerbates EEG spike-wave discharge in children with generalized absence epilepsy: a double-blind controlled study. *Neurology* 1992;42:1000-3.

9) Campbell MB: Neurologic manifestations of allergic disease. *Ann Allergy* 1973;10:485-98.

10) Dengate S, Ruben AJ: Controlled trial of cumulative behavioural effects of a common bread preservative. *Paediatr Child Health* 2002;38:373-6.

11) Dufty, William. *Sugar Blues,* New York, 1975, Warner Books.

12) Feingold BF: Dietary management of nystagmus. *J Neural Transm* 1979;45:107-15.

13) Gerrard JW, Richardson JS, Donat J: Neuropharmacological evaluation of movement disorders that are

adverse reactions to specific foods. *Int J Neurosci* 1994;76:61-9.

14) Geuns JM: Stevioside. *Phytochemistry* 2003;64:913-21.

15) Goldman JA, Lerman RH, Contois JH, Udall JN Jr: Behavioral Effects of Sucrose on Preschool Children. J *Abnorm Child Psychol* 1986;14:565-77.

16) Gregersen S, Jeppesen PB, Holst JJ, Hermansen K: Antihyperglycemic effects of stevioside in type 2 diabetic subjects. *Metabolism* 2004;53:73-6.

17) Jankovic SM: Controversies with aspartame *Med Pregl* 2003;56 Suppl 1:27-9.

18) Kruis W, Forstmaier G, Scheurlen C, Stellaard F: Effects of Diets Low and High in Refined Sugars on Gut Transit, Bile Acid Metabolism and Bacterial Fermentation. *Gut* 1991;32:367-71.

19) Krummel DA, Seligson FH, Guthrie HA: Hyperactivity: is candy causal? *Crit Rev Food Sci Nutr* 1996;36:31-47.

20) Miller JB: *Relief at Last! Neutralization for Food Allergy and Other Illnesses,* 1987, Springfield, IL, Charles C Thomas.

21) Murray JA, Van Dyke C, Plevak MF et al: Trends in the identification and clinical features of celiac disease in a North American community 1950-2001. *Clin Gastroenterol Hepatol* 2003;1:19-27.

22) Olsen DB, Abraham JH: Neuropsychiatric disorders in insulinoma. *Ugeskr Laeger* 1999;161:1420-1.

23) Rippere V: Dietary treatment of chronic obsessional ruminations. *Br J Clin Psychol* 1983;22:314-6.

24) Roberts HJ: Aspartame Disease: A Possible Cause for Concomitant Graves' Disease and Pulmonary Hypertension. *Tex Heart Inst J* 2004;31:105; author reply 105-6.

25) Roberts HJ: *Aspartame (NutraSweet) Is it Safe?* Philadelphia, 1990, Charles Press.

26) Rowe KS, Rowe KJ: Synthetic food coloring and behavior: A dose response effect in a double-blind, placebo-controlled, repeated-measures study. *Journal of Pediatrics* 1994;135:691-8.

27) Santelmann H, Howard JM: Yeast metabolic products, yeast antigens and yeasts as possible triggers for irritable bowel syndrome. *Eur J Gastroenterol Hepatol* 2005;17:21-6.

28) Saxena S, Brody AL, Maidment KM et al: Cerebral glucose metabolism in obsessive-compulsive hoarding. *Am J Psychiatry* 2004;161:1038-48.

29) Schober SE, Sinks TH, Jones RL, Bolger PM et al: Blood mercury levels in US children and women of childbearing age, 1999-2000. *JAMA* 2003;289:667-74.

30) Schwartz JM, Stoessel PW, Baxter LR Jr et al: Systematic changes in cerebral glucose metabolic rate after successful behavior modification treatment of obsessive-compulsive disorder. *Arch Gen Psychiatry* 1996;53:109-13.

31) Simons JP, Rubinstein EN, Kogut VJ, Melfi PJ, Ferguson BJ: Comparison of Multi-Test II skin prick testing to intradermal dilutional testing. *Otolaryngol Head Neck Surg* 2004;130:536-44.

32) Simontacchi CN: *The Crazy Makers: How the Food Industry Is Destroying Our Brains and Harming Our Children,* 2001, Tarcher/Putnam.

33) Speer F: *Handbook of Clinical Allergy,* Boston, London 1982, John Wright.

34) Spiers PA, Sabounjian L, Reiner A, Myers DK et al: Aspartame: neuropsychologic and neurophysiologic evaluation of acute and chronic effects. *Am J Clin Nutr* 1998;68:531-7.

35) Swedo SE, Schapiro MB, Grady CL et al: Cerebral glucose metabolism in childhood-onset obsessive-compulsive disorder. *Arch Gen Psychiatry* 1989;46:518-23.

36) Taylor JP, Krondl MM, Csima AC: Symptom relief and adherence in the rotary diversified diet, a treatment for environmental illness. *Altern Ther Health Med* 2004;10:58-64.

37) Taylor JP, Krondl MM, Csima AC:Assessing adherence to a rotary diversified diet, a treatment for 'environmental illness'. *J Am Diet Assoc* 1998;98:1439-44.

38) Teuber SS, Porch-Curren C: Unproved diagnostic and therapeutic approaches to food allergy and intolerance. *Curr Opin Allergy Clin Immunol* 2003;3:217-21.

39) Uhlig T, Merkenschlager A, Brandmaier R, Egger J: Topographic mapping of brain electrical activity in children with food-induced attention deficit hyperkinetic disorder. *Eur J Pediatr* 1997;156:557-61.

Natural Treatments for Tics & Tourette's

40) Wender EH, Solanto MV: Effects of sugar on aggressive and inattentive behavior in children with attention deficit disorder with hyperactivity and normal children. *Pediatrics* 1991;88:960-6.

41) Wolraich ML, Wilson DB, White JW: The effect of sugar on behavior or cognition in children, A meta-analysis. *JAMA* 1995;274:1617-21.

42) Wurtman RJ, Wurtman jJ, Regan M et al: Effects of normal meals rich in carbohydrates or proteins on plasma tryptophan and tyrosine ratios. *Am J Clin Nutr* 2003;77:128-32.

43) Zelnik N, Pacht A, Obeid R, Lerner A: Range of Neurologic Disorders in Patients with Celiac Disease. *Pediatrics* 2004;113:1672-6.

Chapter 17

1) Adler LA, Rotrosen J, Edson R et al: Vitamin E treatment for tardive dyskinesia. Veterans Affairs Cooperative Study #394 Study Group. *Arch Gen Psychiatry* 1999;56:836-41.

2) Agranoff BW, Fisher SK: Inositol, lithium, and the brain. *Psychopharmacol Bull* 2001;35:5-18.

3) Akhondzadeh S, Mohammadi MR, Khademi M: Zinc sulfate as an adjunct to methylphenidate for the treatment of attention deficit hyperactivity disorder in children: a double blind and randomized trial. *BMC Psychiatry* 2004:8;4:9.

4) Arnold LE: Alternative treatments for adults with attention-deficit hyperactivity disorder (ADHD). *Ann N Y Acad Sci* 2001;931:310-41.

5) Benjamin J. Levine J, Fux M et al: Double-blind, placebo-controlled, crossover trial of inositol treatment for panic disorder. *Am J Psychiatry* 1995;152:1084-6.

6) Baumel S: *Dealing with Depression Naturally*, 2000, Lincolnwood, Illinois, Keats Publishing.

7) Bilici M, Yildirim F et al: Double-blind, placebo-controlled study of zinc sulfate in the treatment of attention deficit hyperactivity disorder. *Prog Neuropsychopharmacol Biol Psychiatry* 2004;28:181-90.

8) Boerner RJ, Klement S: Attenuation of neuroleptic-induced extrapyramidal side effects by Kava special extract WS 1490.*Wien Med Wochenschr* 2004;154:508-10.

9) Chaudhuri PK, Srivastava R, Kumar S et al: Phytotoxic and antimicrobial constituents of Bacopa monnieri and Holmskioldia sanguinea. *Phytother Res* 2004;18:114-7.

10) Chen JR, Hsu SF, Hsu CD, Hwang LH, Yang SC: Dietary patterns and blood fatty acid composition in children with attention-deficit hyperactivity disorder in Taiwan. *J Nutr Biochem* 2004;15:467-72.

11) Clouatre DL: Kava kava: examining new reports of toxicity. *Toxicol Lett* 2004;150:85-96.

12) Cropley M, Cave Z, Ellis J, Middleton RW: Effect of kava and valerian on human physiological and psychological responses to mental stress assessed under laboratory conditions. *Phytother Res* 2002;16:23-7.

13) Das YT, Bagchi M, Bagchi D, Preuss HG: Safety of 5-hydroxy-L-tryptophan. *Toxicol Lett* 2004;150:111-22. Durlach J, Bac P, Bara M, Guiet-Bara A: Physiopathology of symptomatic and latent forms of central nervous hyperexcitability due to magnesium deficiency: a current general scheme. *Magnes Res* 2000;13:293-302.

14) Feingold BF: Dietary management of nystagmus. *J Neural Transm* 1979;45:107-15.

15) Francis AJ, Dempster RJ: Effect of valerian, *Valeriana edulis*, on sleep difficulties in children with intellectual deficits: randomised trial. *Phytomedicine* 2002;9:273-9.

16) Fux M, Levine J, Aviv A et al: Inositol treatment of obsessive-compulsive disorder. *Am J Psychiatry* 1996;153:1219-21.

17) Gastpar M, Singer A, Zeller K: Efficacy and tolerability of hypericum extract STW3 in long-term treatment with a once-daily dosage in comparison with sertraline. *Pharmacopsychiatry* 2005;38:78-86.

18) Gastpar M, Klimm HD: Treatment of anxiety, tension and restlessness states with Kava special extract WS 1490 in general practice: a randomized placebo-controlled double-blind multicenter trial. *Phytomedicine* 2003;10:631-9.

19) Grimaldi BL: The central role of magnesium deficiency in Tourette's syndrome: causal relationships be-

tween magnesium deficiency, altered biochemical pathways and symptoms relating to Tourette's syndrome and several reported comorbid conditions. *Med Hypotheses* 2002;58:47-60.

20) Gruenwald J, Graubaum HJ, Harde A: Effect of a probiotic multivitamin compound on stress and exhaustion. *Adv Ther* 2002;19:141-50.

21) Haddow JE et al: Maternal Thyroid Deficiency During Pregnancy and Subsequent Neuropsychological Development of the Child. *NEJM* 1999;341:549-555.

22) Harding KL, Judah RD, Gant C: Outcome-based comparison of Ritalin versus food-supplement treated children with AD/HD. *Altern Med Rev* 2003;8:319-30.

23) Izzo AA: Drug interactions with St. John's Wort (*Hypericum perforatum*): a review of the clinical evidence. *Int J Clin Pharmacol Ther* 2004;42:139-48.

24) Izzo AA: Herb-drug interactions: an overview of the clinical evidence. *Fundam Clin Pharmacol* 2005;19:1-16.

25) Izzo AA, Ernst E: Interactions between herbal medicines and prescribed drugs: a systematic review. *Drugs* 2001;61:2163-75.

26) Kaplan BJ, Crawford SG, Gardner B, Farrelly G: Treatment of mood lability and explosive rage with minerals and vitamins: two case studies in children. *J Child Adolesc Psychopharmacol* 2002;12:205-19.

27) Konofal E, Lecendreux M, Arnulf I, Mouren MC: Iron deficiency in children with attention-deficit/hyperactivity disorder. *Arch Pediatr Adolesc Med* 2004;158:1113-5.

28) Krystal AD, Ressler I: The use of valerian in neuropsychiatry. *CNS Spectr* 2001;6:841-7.

29) Levine, J, Barak Y, Gonzalves M et al: Double-blind, controlled trial of inositol treatment of depression. *Am J Psychiatry* 1995;152:792-4.

30) Lohr JB, Kuczenski R, Niculescu AB: Oxidative mechanisms and tardive dyskinesia. *CNS Drugs* 2003;17:47-62.

31) Mantel BJ, Meyers A, Tran QY, Rogers S, Jacobson JS: Nutritional supplements and complementary/alternative medicine in Tourette syndrome. *J Child Adolesc Psychopharmacol* 2004;14:582-9.

32) Mauskop A, Altura BT, Cracco RQ, Altura BM: Intravenous magnesium sulfate relieves cluster headaches in patients with low serum ionized magnesium levels. *Headache* 1995;35:597-600.

33) Merchant RE, Andre CA, Sica DA: Nutritional supplementation with Chlorella pyrenoidosa for mild to moderate hypertension. *J Med Food* 2002;5:141-52.

34) Michael N, Sourgens H, Arolt V, Erfurth A: Severe tardive dyskinesia in affective disorders: treatment with vitamin E and C. *Neuropsychobiology* 2002;46 Suppl 1:28-30.

35) Murphy VA, Embrey EC, Rosenberg JM, Smith QR, Rapoport SI: Calcium deficiency enhances cadmium accumulation in the central nervous system. *Brain Res* 1991;557:280-4.

36) Nathan PJ, Clarke J, Lloyd J et al: The acute effects of an extract of Bacopa monniera (Brahmi) on cognitive function in healthy normal subjects. *Hum Psychopharmacol* 2001;16:345-51.

37) Ozcan ME, Gulec M, Ozerol E, Polat R, Akyol O: Antioxidant enzyme activities and oxidative stress in affective disorders. *Int Clin Psychopharmacol* 2004;19:89-95.

38) Palatnik A, Frolov K, Fux M, Benjamin J: Double-blind, controlled, crossover trial of inositol versus fluvoxamine for the treatment of panic disorder. *J Clin Psychopharmacol* 2001;21:335-9.

39) Papakostas GI, Alpert JE, Fava M: S-adenosyl-methionine in depression: a comprehensive review of the literature. *Curr Psychiatry Rep* 2003;5:460-6.

40) Rai D, Bhatia G, Palit G: Adaptogenic effect of Bacopa monniera (Brahmi). *Pharmacol Biochem Behav* 2003;75:823-30.

41) Ravikumar A, Deepadevi KV, Arun P, Manojkumar V, Kurup PA: Tryptophan and tyrosine catabolic pattern in neuropsychiatric disorders. *Neurol India* 2000;48:231-8.

42) Richardso AJ, Puri BK: A randomized double-blind, placebo-controlled study of the effects of supplementation with highly unsaturated fatty acids on ADHD-related symptoms in children with specific learning difficulties. *Prog Neuropsychopharmacol Biol Psychiatry* 2002;26:233-9.

43) Rippere V: Dietary treatment of chronic obsessional ruminations. *Br J Clin Psychol* 1983;22:314-6.

Natural Treatments for Tics & Tourette's

44) Roodenrys S, Booth D, Bulzomi S et al: Chronic effects of Brahmi (Bacopa monniera) on human memory. *Neuropsychopharmacology* 2002;27:279-81.

45) Sandyk R: L-tryptophan in neuropsychiatric disorders: a review. *Int J Neurosci* 1992;67:127-44.

46) Soares KV, McGrath JJ: Vitamin E for neuroleptic-induced tardive dyskinesia. *Cochrane Database Syst Rev* 2001;CD000209.

47) Stough C, Lloyd J, Clarke J et al: The chronic effects of an extract of Bacopa monniera (Brahmi) on cognitive function in healthy human subjects. *Psychopharmacology* 2001;156:481-4.

48) Swedo SE, Pietrini P, Leonard HL et al: Cerebral glucose metabolism in childhood-onset obsessive-compulsive disorder. Revisualization during pharmacotherapy. *Arch Gen Psychiatry* 1992;49:690-4.

49) Van Oudheusden LJ, Scholte HR: Efficacy of carnitine in the treatment of children with attention-deficit hyperactivity disorder. *Prostaglandins Leukot Essent Fatty Acids.* 2002;67:33-8.

50) Walsh WJ, Glab LB, Haakenson ML: Reduced violent behavior following biochemical therapy. *Physiol Behav* 2004;82:835-9.

51) Wender EH, Solanto MV: Effects of sugar on aggressive and inattentive behavior in children with attention deficit disorder with hyperactivity and normal children. *Pediatrics* 1991;88:960-6.

52) Wheatley D: Stress-induced insomnia treated with kava and valerian: singly and in combination. *Hum Psychopharmacol* 2001;16:353-6.

53) Wood JL, Allison RG: Effects of consumption of choline and lecithin on neurological and cardiovascular systems. *Fed Proc* 1982;41:3015-21.

54) Wurtman RJ: Nutrients affecting brain composition and behavior. *Integr Psychiatry* 1987; 226-38; discussion 238-57.

55) Wurtman RJ: Stress and the adrenocortical control of epinephrine synthesis. *Metabolism* 2002;51:11-4.

56) Zhang XY, Zhou DF, Cao LY et al: The effect of vitamin E treatment on tardive dyskinesia and blood superoxide dismutase: a double-blind placebo-controlled trial. *J Clin Psychopharmacol* 2004;24:83-6.

57) Zinner, S: Tourette syndrome: Much more than tics—part 1. *Contemporary Pediatrics* 2004;21,29.

Chapter 20

1) Miltenberger RG, Fuqua RW: A comparison of contingent vs non-contingent competing response practice in the treatment of nervous habits. *J Behav Ther Exp Psychiatr* 2985;16:195-200.

2) Azrin NH, Peterson AL: Habit reversal for the treatment of Tourette Syndrome. *Behav Res Ther* 1988;26:347-51.

3) Azrin NH, Peterson AL: Treatment of Tourette Syndrome by habit reversal: A waiting-list control group comparison. *Behav Ther* 1990; 21:301-18.

4) Chanksy, Tamar E: *Freeing Your Child from Obsessive-Compulsive Disorder : A Powerful, Practical Program for Parents of Children and Adolescent*s, 2001, New York, Three Rivers Press.

5) Chanksy, Tamar E: *Freeing Your Child from Anxiety: Powerful, Practical Solutions to Overcome Your Child's Fears, Worries, and Phobias*, 2004, New York, Broadway Books.

6) Culbertson FM: A four-step hypnotherapy model for Gilles de la Tourette's syndrome. *Am J Clin Hypn* 1989;31:252-6.

7) Miltenberger RG, Fuqua RW, Woods DW: Applying behavior analysis to clinical problems: Review and analysis of habit reversal. *J Appl Behav Anal* 1998;31:447-469.

8) Peterson AL, Campise RL, Azrin NH: Behavioral and pharmacological treatments for tic and habit disorders: A review. *J Dev Behav Pediatr* 1994;15:430-441.

9) O'Connor KP, Brault M, Robillard S et al: Evaluation of a cognitive-behavioural program for the management of chronic tic and habit disorders. *Behav Res Ther* 2001;39:667-681.

10) Wilhelm S, Deckersbach T, Coffey BJ, Bohne A Peterson AL, Baer L: Habit reversal versus supportive psychotherapy for Tourette's disorder: A randomized controlled trial. *Am J Psychiatry* 2003;160:1175-7.

Chapter 21

1) Carlson LE, Ursuliak Z, Goodey E, Angen M, Speca M: The effects of a mindfulness meditation-based stress reduction program on mood and symptoms of stress in cancer outpatients: 6-month follow-up. *Support Care Cancer* 2001; 112-23.

2) Croxford JL, Yamamura T: Cannabinoids and the immune system: Potential for the treatment of inflammatory diseases? *J Neuroimmunol* 2005 Sep;166(1-2):3-18

3) Elster, EL: Upper Cervical Chiropractic Care for a Nine-Year-Old Male with Tourette Syndrome, Attention Deficit Hyperactivity Disorder, Depression, Asthma, Insomnia, and Headaches: A Case Report. *J Vertebral Subluxation Res* 2003;4.

4) Factor SA, Molho ES: Adult-onset tics associated with peripheral injury. *Mov Disord* 1997;12:1052-5.

5) Field T, Ironson G, Scafidi F et al: Massage therapy reduces anxiety and enhances EEG pattern of alertness and math computations. *Int J Neurosci* 1996;86:197-205.

6) Frei H, Everts R, von Ammon K et al: Homeopathic treatment of children with attention deficit hyperactivity disorder: a randomised, double blind, placebo controlled crossover trial. *Eur J Pediatr* 2005; [E-pub ahead of print].

7) Hammond DC: Neurofeedback with anxiety and affective disorders. *Child Adolesc Psychiatr Clin N Am* 2005;14:105-23.

8) Huizink AC, Mulder EJ: Maternal smoking, drinking or cannabis use during pregnancy and neurobehavioral and cognitive functioning in human offspring. *Neurosci Biobehav Rev* 2005; Advance E-publication

9) Jorm AF, Christensen H, Griffiths KM et al: Effectiveness of complementary and self-help treatments for anxiety disorders. *Med J Aust* 2004;181:S29-46.

10) Kabat-Zinn J, Massion AO, Kristeller J et al: Effectiveness of a meditation-based stress reduction program in the treatment of anxiety disorders. *Am J Psychiatry* 1992;149:936-43.

11) Khilnani S, Field T, Hernandez-Reif M, Schanberg S: Massage therapy improves mood and behavior of students with attention-deficit/hyperactivity disorder. *Adolescence* 2003;38:623-38.

12) King WP, Motes JM: The intracutaneous progressive dilution multi-food test. *Otolaryngol Head Neck Surg* 1991;104:235-8.

13) Kostanecka-Endress T, Banaschewski T, Kinkelbur J et al: Disturbed sleep in children with Tourette syndrome: a polysomnographic study *J Psychosom Res* 2003;55:23-9.

14) Krauss JK, Jankovic J: Tics secondary to craniocerebral trauma. *Mov Disord* 1997;12:776-82.

15) Monastra VJ, Lynn S, Linden M et al: Electroencephalographic biofeedback in the treatment of attention-deficit/hyperactivity disorder. *Appl Psychophysiol Biofeedback* 2005;30:95-114.

16) Majumdar A, Appleton RE: Delayed and severe but transient Tourette syndrome after head injury. *Pediatr Neurol* 2002;27:314-7.

17) Majumdar M, Grossman P, Dietz-Waschkowski B, Kersig S, Walach H: Does mindfulness meditation contribute to health? Outcome evaluation of a German sample. *J Altern Complement Med* 2002;8:719-30.

18) Moore NC: A review of EEG biofeedback treatment of anxiety disorders. *Clin Electroencephalogr* 2000;31:1-6.

19) Moran RW, Gibbons P: Intraexaminer and interexaminer reliability for palpation of the cranial rhythmic impulse at the head and sacrum. *J Manipulative Physiol Ther* 2001;24:183-90.

20) Passalacqua G, Compalati E, Schiappoli M, Senna G: Complementary and alternative medicine for the treatment and diagnosis of asthma and allergic diseases. *Monaldi Arch Chest Dis* 2005;63:47-54.

21) Plotkin BJ, Rodos JJ, Kappler R et al: Adjunctive osteopathic manipulative treatment in women with depression: a pilot study. *J Am Osteopath Assoc* 2001;101:517-23.

22) Rojas NL, Chan E: Old and new controversies in the alternative treatment of attention-deficit hyperactivity disorder. *Ment Retard Dev Disabil Res Rev* 2005;11(2):116-30.

23) Schmitt WH Jr, Leisman G: Correlation of applied kinesiology muscle testing findings with serum immunoglobulin levels for food allergies. *Int J Neurosci* 1998;96:237-44.

24) Singer C, Snachez-Ramos J, Weiner WJ: A case of post-traumatic tic disorder. *Mov Disord* 1989;4:342-4.

25) Singh, Rajinder: *Inner and Outer Peace through Meditation,* 2003, HarperCollins Publishers.

26) Sterman MB: Basic concepts and clinical findings in the treatment of seizure disorders with EEG operant conditioning. *Clin Electroencephalogr* 2000;31:45-55.

27) Tansey MA: A simple and a complex tic (Gilles de la Tourette's syndrome): their response to EEG sensorimotor rhythm biofeedback training. *Int J Psychophysiol* 1986;4:91-7.

28) Witt C, Keil T, Selim D et al: Outcome and costs of homoeopathic and conventional treatment strategies: A comparative cohort study in patients with chronic disorders. *Complement Ther Med* 2005;13:79-86.

29) Wu L, Li H, Kang L: 156 cases of Gilles de la Tourette's syndrome treated by acupuncture. *J Tradit Chin Med* 1996;16:211-3.

Afterword

1) Brody, J: The Tics of Tourette's Often Go Undiagnosed. *New York Times*, January 18, 2005.

2) Zinner, S: Tourette syndrome: Much more than tics—part 2. *Contemporary Pediatrics* 2004;21,39.

INDEX

About the Author

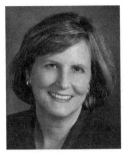

Sheila J. Rogers, MS, is a leading educator in the field of integrative and complementary approaches to neurologic disorders. She is founder and director of the international nonprofit organization Association for Comprehensive NeuroTherapy (ACN), and editor of Latitudes Online, a magazine featuring natural therapies for autism, obsessive-compulsive disorder, depression, anxiety, attention deficit disorders, tic disorders/Tourette syndrome, and learning problems. Also a private consultant, Rogers serves on the advisory board for Health Journal Television, hosted by General Alexander Haig.